Neonatal Nursing

Editor

BETH C. DIEHL

CRITICAL CARE
NURSING CLINICS
OF NORTH AMERICA

www.ccnursing.theclinics.com

Consulting Editor
JAN FOSTER

December 2018 • Volume 30 • Number 4

ELSEVIER

1600 John F. Kennedy Boulevard • Suite 1800 • Philadelphia, Pennsylvania, 19103-2899

http://www.theclinics.com

CRITICAL CARE NURSING CLINICS OF NORTH AMERICA Volume 30, Number 4
December 2018 ISSN 0899-5885, ISBN-13: 978-0-323-64331-3

Editor: Kerry Holland
Developmental Editor: Laura Fisher

Critical Care Nursing Clinics of North America (ISSN 0899-5885) is published quarterly by Elsevier Inc., 360 Park Avenue South, New York, NY 10010-1710. Months of issue are March, June, September, and December. Business and Editorial Offices: 1600 John F. Kennedy Blvd., Suite 1800, Philadelphia, PA 19103-2899. Periodicals postage paid at New York, NY and additional mailing offices. Subscription prices are $155.00 per year for US individuals, $385.00 per year for US institutions, $100.00 per year for US students and residents, $200.00 per year for Canadian individuals, $483.00 per year for Canadian institutions, $230.00 per year for international individuals, $483.00 per year for international institutions and $115.00 per year for Canadian and international students/residents. To receive student/resident rate, orders must be accompanied by name of affiliated institution, data of term, and the *signature* of program/residency coordinator on institution letterhead. Orders will be billed at individual rate until proof of status is received. Foreign air speed delivery is included in all *Clinics* subscription prices. All prices are subject to change without notice. **POSTMASTER:** Send address changes to *Critical Care Nursing Clinics of North America*, Elsevier Health Sciences Division, Subscription Customer Service, 3251 Riverport Lane, Maryland Heights, MO 63043. **Customer Service: 1-800-654-2452 (US and Canada); 314-447-8871 (outside US and Canada). Fax: 314-447-8029. E-mail:** JournalsCustomerService-usa@elsevier.com **(for print support) and** JournalsOnlineSupport-usa@elsevier.com **(for online support).**

Reprints. For copies of 100 or more of articles in this publication, please contact the Commercial Reprints Department, Elsevier Inc., 360 Park Avenue South, New York, New York, 10010-1710; Tel.: 212-633-3874, Fax: 212-633-3820, and E-mail: reprints@elsevier.com.

Critical Care Nursing Clinics of North America is covered in *MEDLINE/PubMed (Index Medicus), International Nursing Index, Nursing Citation Index, Cumulative Index to Nursing and Allied Health Literature, and RNdex Top 100.*

Contributors

CONSULTING EDITOR

JAN FOSTER, PhD, APRN, CNS
Formerly, Associate Professor, College of Nursing, Texas Woman's University, Houston, Texas; Currently, President, Nursing Inquiry and Intervention, Inc, The Woodlands, Texas

EDITOR

BETH C. DIEHL, DNP, NNP-BC, CCRN, LNCC
Neonatal Nurse Practitioner, Transport Nurse, The Johns Hopkins Hospital, Maryland Regional Neonatal Transport Program, Charlotte R. Bloomberg Children's Center, Baltimore, Maryland

AUTHORS

LESLIE ALTIMIER, DNP, RN, MSN, NE-BC
Affiliate Associate Professor, Northeastern University, Boston, Massachusetts; Director of Clinical Research & Innovation, Philips Health Tech, Cambridge, Massachusetts

LYNN E. BAYNE, PhD, APRN, NNP-BC
Neonatal Nurse Practitioner, Christiana Care Health System, Newark, Delaware; Alfred I. duPont Hospital for Children, Wilmington, Delaware

JIE CHEN, BS, MSN, RN
School of Nursing, University of Connecticut, Storrs, Connecticut

XIAOMEI S. CONG, PhD, RN
Director, Center for Advancement in Managing Pain, Associate Professor, School of Nursing, University of Connecticut, Storrs, Connecticut

BETH C. DIEHL, DNP, NNP-BC, CCRN, LNCC
Neonatal Nurse Practitioner, Transport Nurse, The Johns Hopkins Hospital, Maryland Regional Neonatal Transport Program, Charlotte R. Bloomberg Children's Center, Baltimore, Maryland

KAREN DITTMAN, MSN, CRNP, NNP-BC
Neonatal Nurse Practitioner, Neonatal Intensive Care Unit, The Johns Hopkins Hospital, Charlotte R. Bloomberg Children's Center, Baltimore, Maryland

KAREN M. FRANK, DNP, RNC-NIC, APRN-CNS
Clinical Associate Professor, Department of Nursing, Towson University, Towson, Maryland

EMORY FRY, MD
Chief Executive Officer, Cognitive Medical Systems, Inc, San Diego, California

SHEILA M. GEPHART, PhD, RN
Community and Health Systems Science, Associate Professor, College of Nursing, The University of Arizona, Tucson, Arizona

SHAWN HUGHES, BS, RRT-NPS, CPFT
Neonatal Clinical Coordinator, NICU Respiratory Care Services, Neonatal Intensive Care Unit, The Johns Hopkins Hospital, Charlotte R. Bloomberg Children's Center, Baltimore, Maryland

STEPHANIE HUGHES, RN, BSN
Nurse Clinician III, Neonatal Intensive Care Unit, The Johns Hopkins Hospital, Charlotte R. Bloomberg Children's Center, Baltimore, Maryland

KRISTINE A. KARLSEN, PhD, APRN, NNP-BC
Author and Program Director, The S.T.A.B.L.E. Program, Park City, Utah; Neonatal Nurse Practitioner, Intermountain Healthcare, Primary Children's Hospital, Intermountain Medical Center, Salt Lake City, Utah

NANCY J. MACMULLEN, PhD, APN/CNS, RNC, HR-OB, CNE
Chairperson/Director, Department of Nursing, Governors State University, University Park, Illinois

EMILY F. MOORE, RN, MSN, CPNP
Nurse Practitioner, Regional Cardiology Program, Seattle Children's Hospital, Seattle, Washington; Robert Wood Johnson Foundation Future of Nursing Scholar, University of Arizona College of Nursing, Tucson, Arizona

MALLORY PERRY, BSN, MS, RN, CPN
School of Nursing, University of Connecticut, Storrs, Connecticut

RAYLENE PHILLIPS, MD, MA, FAAP, FABM, IBCLC
Associate Professor of Pediatrics, Division of Neonatology, Loma Linda University School of Medicine, Director of Neonatal Neurodevelopment, Loma Linda University Children's Hospital, Loma Linda, California; Director of Neonatal Services, Loma Linda University Medical Center - Murrieta, Murrieta, California

MARY L. PUCHALSKI, DNP, APRN, CNS, NNP-BC
Neonatal Nurse Practitioner, Ann & Robert H. Lurie Children's Hospital of Chicago, Clinical Assistant Professor, NNP-DNP Program Director, Department of Women, Children and Family Health Sciences, College of Nursing, The University of Illinois at Chicago, Chicago, Illinois

YVETTE PUGH, MS, CRNP, NNP-BC
Neonatal Nurse Practitioner, Department of Pediatrics, Community Neonatal Associates, Holy Cross Hospital, Silver Spring, Maryland

TERRI L. RUSSELL, DNP, APRN, NNP-BC
Neonatal Nurse Practitioner, Ann & Robert H. Lurie Children's Hospital of Chicago, Clinical Assistant Professor, Department of Women, Children and Family Health Sciences, College of Nursing, The University of Illinois at Chicago, Chicago, Illinois

LINDA F. SAMSON, PhD, RN, BC, NEA, BC
Professor, Department of Nursing, Governors State University, University Park, Illinois

ELIZABETH A. SCHUMP, MSN, ARNP, NNP-BC
Overland Park Regional Medical Center, NICU, Overland Park, Kansas

ZEWEN TAN
Undergraduate Honors Student, Department of Molecular and Cell Biology, School of Medicine, School of Nursing, University of Connecticut, Storrs, Connecticut

TESSA WEIDIG
Undergraduate Honors Student, School of Nursing, University of Connecticut, Storrs, Connecticut

JULIE E. WILLIAMS, MS, CRNP, NNP-BC
Neonatal Nurse Practitioner, Department of Neonatology, The Johns Hopkins Hospital, Baltimore, Maryland

WANLI XU, BS, MS, RN
School of Nursing, University of Connecticut, Storrs, Connecticut

JEANETTE G. ZAICHKIN, RN, MN, NNP-BC
Owner, Positive Pressure, PLLC, Tacoma, Washington

Contents

Erratum xiii

Preface: Neonatal Nursing: Clinical Concepts and Practice Implications xv

Beth C. Diehl

The Late Preterm: A Population at Risk 431

Julie E. Williams and Yvette Pugh

Late preterm infants (LPIs) are born between 34 0/7 and 36 6/7 weeks' gestation and account for 72% of all preterm births in the United States. Born as much as 6 weeks early, the LPI misses the critical growth and development specific to the third trimester. The loss of this critical period leaves the LPI physiologically and metabolically immature and prone to various morbidities. Common morbidities include respiratory complications, feeding difficulty, hypoglycemia, temperature instability, hyperbilirubinemia, and neurodevelopmental delays.

Increased Nursing Participation in Multidisciplinary Rounds to Enhance Communication, Patient Safety, and Parent Satisfaction 445

Karen Dittman and Stephanie Hughes

Effective communication among health care team members is a mainstay of patient safety, especially in a neonatal ICU (NICU), given small errors can have serious and life-threating consequences. Ineffective communication with families of hospitalized children can lead to decreased satisfaction and trust in the health care team. To enhance communication, the NICU nursing staff at the Johns Hopkins Children's Center spearheaded an initiative to create an enhanced nursing role in multidisciplinary patient rounds. Education of the nursing staff and other team members and the development of a rounding script for nurses was instrumental for successful implementation.

Standardized Feeding Protocols to Reduce Risk of Necrotizing Enterocolitis in Fragile Infants Born Premature or with Congenital Heart Disease: Implementation Science Needed 457

Sheila M. Gephart, Emily F. Moore, and Emory Fry

Although a unit-adopted standardized feeding protocol (SFP) for neonates is standard of care, implementation strategies for SFPs vary across neonatal and pediatric intensive care. Besides improving growth and reducing feeding interruptions, SFPs reduce risk for necrotizing enterocolitis in infants with heart disease or born premature. The purpose of this article is to bridge the gap between recommended and actual care using SFPs.

Neonatal Hypoglycemia: Is There a Sweet Spot? **467**

Mary L. Puchalski, Terri L. Russell, and Kristine A. Karlsen

Hypoglycemia is one of the most common neonatal problems. Despite increasing evidence that hypoglycemia is linked to neurologic impairment, knowledge regarding the specific value or duration of hypoglycemia that results in injury to the brain remains unclear. Current published statements/guidelines focused on preventing clinically significant hypoglycemia are conflicting and continue to be based on low evidence. This article reviews transitional events leading to extrauterine euglycemia, risk factors contributing to transient or persistent hypoglycemia, and common treatment approaches. Current information related to neurodevelopmental outcomes and screening strategies to prevent significant hypoglycemia with early treatment is described.

Big Data in Neonatal Health Care: Big Reach, Big Reward? **481**

Lynn E. Bayne

Analog-to-digital data conversion has created massive amounts of historical and real-time health care data. Costs associated with neonatal health issues are high. Big data use in the neonatal intensive care unit has the potential to facilitate earlier detection of clinical deterioration, expedite application of efficient clinical decision-making algorithms based on real-time and historical data mining, and yield significant cost-savings.

Fetal Surgery and Delayed Cord Clamping: Neonatal Implications **499**

Karen M. Frank

Advances made in the last several decades in the care of the fetus and newborn have had a significant impact on morbidity and mortality. Delayed umbilical cord clamping in the preterm newborn results in fewer transfusions for anemia, decreased intraventricular hemorrhage, and decreased necrotizing enterocolitis. Because of advances made in fetal ultrasound diagnosis and technological advances, fetal surgeries to treat congenital diaphragmatic hernia, myelomeningocele, twin-to-twin transfusion syndrome, fetal lower urinary tract obstructions, amniotic band syndrome, and congenital cystic adenoid malformation or congenital pulmonary airway malformations have improved the quality of life and survival for these patients.

Neonatal Encephalopathy: Current Management and Future Trends **509**

Elizabeth A. Schump

It is well-documented in the literature that infants who suffer from hypoxic ischemic encephalopathy are at high risk for neurologic sequelae or even death. With the addition of therapeutic hypothermia into the treatment regimen for neonatal hypoxic ischemic encephalopathy, newborns afflicted with hypoxic ischemic encephalopathy were given the opportunity for a better outcome. Questions linger as to the most optimal treatment strategy of therapeutic hypothermia for these newborns. The goal of this article is to discuss current management strategies, as well as future trends, for infants with hypoxic ischemic encephalopathy.

Modes of Neonatal Ventilation: Breathe Deeply! 523

Shawn Hughes

The art and science of neonatal ventilation continue to evolve with advances in technology and as a result of evidenced based research. Although some historically administered therapies remain such as nasal continuous positive airway pressure, newer therapies have emerged in the neonatal intensive care unit such as pressure regulated volume control and neurally adjusted ventilatory assist. The challenge for clinicians continues to be which mode will support the patient's medical diagnosis with minimal barotrauma or lung injury. Vigilance and collaborative discussions among the treatment team remain the cornerstones of respiratory care practice parameters in the neonatal intensive care environment.

Neonatal Resuscitation: Neonatal Resuscitation Program 7th Edition Practice Integration 533

Jeanette G. Zaichkin

The Neonatal Resuscitation Program meets the education and training needs of health care professionals in the United States who manage newborn resuscitation in hospitals. The Neonatal Resuscitation Program focuses on cognitive, technical, and behavioral skills. This article briefly describes the preparation and principles of newborn resuscitation and selected components of the Neonatal Resuscitation Program Flow Diagram. Five resuscitation scenarios of increasing complexity are used to illustrate how the guidelines are integrated into clinical practice.

Neonatal Pain: Perceptions and Current Practice 549

Mallory Perry, Zewen Tan, Jie Chen, Tessa Weidig, Wanli Xu, and Xiaomei S. Cong

Neonates may experience more than 300 painful procedures throughout their hospitalizations. Prior to 1980, there was a longstanding misconception that neonates do not experience pain. Current studies demonstrate that not only do neonates experience pain but also, due to their immature nervous systems, they are hypersensitive to painful stimuli. Poorly treated pain may lead to negative long-term consequences. Proper assessment of neonate pain is vital. The use of nonpharmacologic treatments may be beneficial in alleviating neonate pain. Pharmacologic treatments in the neonate have been well established. Pharmacologic and nonpharmacologic interventions can be used in conjunction to increase the efficacy of analgesia.

Neuroprotective Care of Extremely Preterm Infants in the First 72 Hours After Birth 563

Leslie Altimier and Raylene Phillips

Birth at extremely low gestational ages presents a significant threat to infants' survival, health, development, and future well-being. After birth, a critical period of brain development must continue outside the womb. Neuro-supportive and neuroprotective family centered developmental care for and standardized care practices for extremely preterm infants have been shown to improve outcomes. Neuroprotective interventions must include a focus on the emotional connections of infants and their families. Being in skin-to-skin contact with the mother is the developmentally expected environment for all mammals and is especially important for supporting physiologic stability and neurodevelopment of preterm infants.

Neonatal Abstinence Syndrome: An Uncontrollable Epidemic **585**

Nancy J. MacMullen and Linda F. Samson

There is an uncontrollable epidemic of drug abuse, with the misuse of opioids the most alarming. Along with the increase in opioid abuse, there exists a concomitant upsurge in the number of neonates experiencing neonatal abstinence syndrome (NAS) due to the effects of the mother's withdrawal from the drug. Neonates experiencing NAS exhibit various nervous system, gastrointestinal, and respiratory untoward symptoms. Diagnosis is determined by taking an accurate maternal history and assessment of clinical signs and symptoms. Clinical management strategies include pharmacologic and nonpharmacologic therapies. Nursing care is evidence based, includes nonpharmacologic therapies, and focuses on prevention and support.

Neonatal Transport: Current Trends and Practices **597**

Beth C. Diehl

Since the inception of organized neonatal transport in the 1940s, advances in clinical care and technology have made the neonatal intensive care unit even more mobile in terms of care delivery. There currently exists an emphasis on quality metrics and simulation-based training for transport team members to achieve high levels of individual and team competence. Emerging therapies such as active cooling for neuroprotective hypothermia and high-frequency ventilation provide evidence-based care in the transport environment to enhance clinical outcomes. Accreditation of neonatal transport programs is now embraced as an indicator of competency and compliance with transport standards.

CRITICAL CARE NURSING CLINICS OF NORTH AMERICA

FORTHCOMING ISSUES

March 2019
Interventions for Cardiovascular Disease
Leanne H. Fowler and Jessica Landry, *Editors*

June 2019
Quality Outcomes and Costs
Deborah Garbee and Denise Danna, *Editors*

September 2019
Cardiothoracic Surgical Critical Care
Bryan Boling, *Editor*

RECENT ISSUES

September 2018
Sepsis
Jennifer B. Martin and Jennifer E. Badeaux, *Editors*

June 2018
Human Factors and Technology in the ICU
Shu-Fen Wung, *Editor*

March 2018
Gastrointestinal Issues and Complications
Deborah Weatherspoon and Debra Henline Sullivan, *Editors*

SERIES OF RELATED INTEREST

Nursing Clinics of North America
http://www.nursing.theclinics.com

Erratum

The article "Etomidate as an Induction Agent in Sepsis" by Raymond J. Devlin and David Kalil was mistakenly omitted from the September 2018 issue of *Critical Care Nursing Clinics* (Vol. 30, Issue 3) due to a production error. This article is now available via our website at: https://www.ccnursing.theclinics.com/.

For citing this article, please use the following reference: Devlin RJ, Kalil D. Etomidate as an induction agent in sepsis. *Crit Care Nurs Clin North Am*. 2018;30(3):e1-e9.

Crit Care Nurs Clin N Am 30 (2018) xiii
https://doi.org/10.1016/j.cnc.2018.10.001

Preface

Neonatal Nursing: Clinical Concepts and Practice Implications

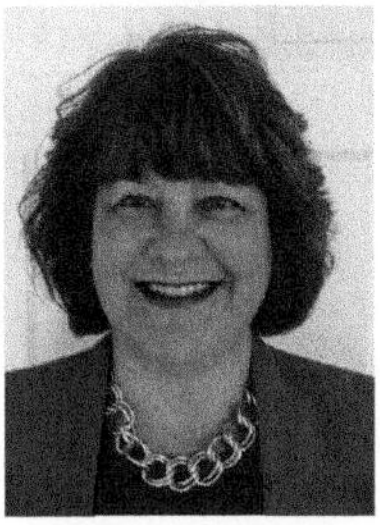

Beth C. Diehl, DNP, NNP-BC, CCRN, LNCC
Editor

From the birth of "modern" neonatal intensive care nursing in the 1960s to the 1970s until present day, an evolution in practice has occurred related to a multitude of factors. Certainly, evidence-based practice initiatives coupled with technological advances and changes in pharmacologic regimens continue to alter day-to-day management in neonatal intensive care units (NICU) across the United States. As neonatal nurses and other medical professionals strive to deliver high-quality care, it is imperative that collective experiences and research be shared across the profession in peer-reviewed literature and other reference materials.

The most recent publication of the neonatal-based *Nursing Clinics of North America* issue was in 2009, which seems ancient in terms of the practice and care delivery changes that have taken place in the interim. For example, therapeutic hypothermia has now become a mainstay for the treatment and management of neonatal encephalopathy since the cooling studies were begun in the early to mid 2000s. Although high-frequency ventilation has been an integral component of respiratory care in the NICU environment for many years, the ability to provide that mode of ventilation during transport is fairly recent related to the availability of commercial equipment. In addition, the American Academy of Pediatrics has since redefined levels of perinatal care. The previous three-level model delineation has now been changed to a four-level system of care delivery. The Neonatal Resuscitation Program, which outlines delivery room management for the over 4 million neonates born annually in the United States, published new guidelines in both 2011 (6th edition) and 2017 (7th edition). Other topics of rapid progression related to ongoing research include the management of neonatal hypoglycemia, assessment and treatment of pain, and the integration of delayed cord clamping at the time of delivery into care algorithms. More importantly, the existence of the

Crit Care Nurs Clin N Am 30 (2018) xv–xvi
https://doi.org/10.1016/j.cnc.2018.09.001
0899-5885/18/© 2018 Published by Elsevier Inc.

electronic medical record and resultant access to large data sets allow for care delivery to be more closely assessed and scrutinized as a driver for high-level outcomes. As the nation endures an opioid epidemic, the management of neonates experiencing intrauterine drug exposure and subsequent withdrawal has posed challenges for the multidisciplinary care team not only for effective and therapeutic in-patient care but also for discharge planning. These are but a few of the many changes that have occurred over the course of the last ten years.

This issue provides a comprehensive overview and update of clinical practice modifications, policy initiatives, and protocol alterations for the neonatal care provider so that outcomes can continue to be optimized. The smallest and most critically ill neonates in America will continue to demand a highly skilled and competent care team. Nursing is an integral component of that team and has been at the forefront by embracing and integrating these changes into practice and will continue to do so in the years to come.

Beth C. Diehl, DNP, NNP-BC, CCRN, LNCC
The Johns Hopkins Hospital
Maryland Regional Neonatal Transport Program
Charlotte R. Bloomberg Children's Center
1800 Orleans Street, Room 8547
Baltimore, MD 21287, USA

E-mail address:
Bdiehls1@jhmi.edu

The Late Preterm

A Population at Risk

Julie E. Williams, MS, CRNP, NNP-BC[a,*], Yvette Pugh, MS, CRNP, NNP-BC[b]

KEYWORDS

- Late preterm infant • Respiratory complications • Hypoglycemia • Neonatal nutrition
- Hyperbilirubinemia • Neonatal morbidity • Neurodevelopmental outcomes

KEY POINTS

- The most common morbidities experienced by the late preterm infant include respiratory complications, feeding difficulty, hypoglycemia, temperature instability, hyperbilirubinemia, and neurodevelopmental delays.
- The late preterm infant has a higher morbidity and mortality rate compared with their term counterparts.
- Discharge planning and follow-up care is crucial for reducing hospital readmission rates and promoting healthy growth and development.

INTRODUCTION

Late preterm infants (LPIs) are born between 34 0/7 and 36 6/7 weeks gestational age. From 2014 to 2016, the LPI birth rate rose from 6.82% to 7.09%, accounting for approximately 72% of all preterm births in the United States.[1] The increase in preterm births, has been attributed to the rise in assisted reproductive therapy, improved obstetric surveillance, multiple births, and maternal factors, including advanced maternal age.[2] LPIs are usually larger than premature infants and often mistakenly equated to the term infant. Although they may be close to term, the loss of the last 6 weeks of gestation is vital to their physiologic and metabolic maturity. Because of their physiologic and metabolic immaturity, they have higher morbidity and mortality rates compared with term infants (gestational age $\geq$37 weeks).[3]

Research has shown that the newborn morbidity rate doubles for every gestational week less than 38 weeks.[4] For LPIs, this translates to a morbidity rate as high as 51% in the 34-week infant.[3] LPIs experience higher morbidities during hospitalization and higher readmission rates during their first year of life when compared with the term

Disclosure Statement: The authors have nothing to disclose.
[a] Department of Neonatology, The Johns Hopkins Hospital, The Charlotte R. Bloomberg Children Center Building, 1800 Orleans Street, Baltimore, MD 21287, USA; [b] Department of Pediatrics, Community Neonatal Associates, Holy Cross Hospital, 1500 Forest Glen Road, Silver Spring, MD 20910, USA
* Corresponding author.
E-mail address: jewilliams2@outlook.com

Crit Care Nurs Clin N Am 30 (2018) 431–443
https://doi.org/10.1016/j.cnc.2018.07.001 ccnursing.theclinics.com

infant.[2,5] The most common morbidities experienced include respiratory complications, feeding difficulty, hypoglycemia, temperature instability, hyperbilirubinemia, and neurodevelopmental delays.[6–8] Given the heightened risks LPIs are exposed to, this article presents an overview of the complications placing them at risk for increased morbidity, mortality, and long-term adverse outcomes (**Table 1**).

RESPIRATORY COMPLICATIONS

LPIs have a higher incidence and risk of respiratory complications than the term infant. Respiratory complications more commonly encountered include respiratory distress syndrome (RDS), transient tachypnea of the newborn (TTN), and apnea.[5,9] LPIs are born during the saccular and alveolar stages of lung development. These stages of development are characterized by the development and remodeling of the respiratory bronchioles and alveoli, which are important for the process of surfactant synthesis and secretion, and gas exchange.[10,11] An interruption in this development leads to a delay in lung maturation and predisposes the LPI to RDS. Other factors, including the ineffective clearance of fetal lung fluid during the transition to neonatal life, can diminish alveolar gas exchange and is often implicated in TTN.[12] Compounding factors including Cesarean birth without the benefit of labor, and maternal and/or fetal complications contribute to the increased incidence of RDS, TTN, and apnea.

In a large retrospective study, found infants born at 34 weeks' gestation required more oxygen supplementation and delivery of oxygen via bag-mask ventilation in the delivery room than infants born at each advancing week of gestation until 39 weeks.[5] Among this LPI population, RDS was the most common respiratory morbidity followed by TTN. When morbidities were compared across gestational ages, the adjusted odds ratio for RDS and TTN decreased from 34 to 38 weeks' gestation.[13] In another retrospective cross-sectional study, 39.4% of all LPIs admitted to the neonatal intensive care unit (NICU) were admitted for respiratory distress, making this the number one reason for admission. Within this cohort, 34.4% were diagnosed with TTN, 4.4% with pneumonia, and 0.8% with meconium aspiration syndrome.[2]

The incidence of central, obstructive, and mixed apnea is higher in the LPI than the term infant. The etiology of apnea is multifactorial, reflecting an immature neurologic system and the physiologic immaturity of the respiratory system. Preterm infants have a decreased ventilatory response to increased carbon dioxide levels and a biphasic ventilatory response to hypoxia.[14] The very compliant chest wall and upper airway of the preterm infant also plays a role in the propensity toward apnea.[13,15] The incidence of apnea within the literature has varied based on the definition, acquisition, and documentation clarity of the event. In a meta-analysis of studies, the incidence of apnea to be 0.9% in the LPI and 0.05% in the term infant.[14] A decrease in apnea was observed with increasing gestational age. LPIs can also experience apnea associated with feedings because of a lack of coordination among sucking, swallowing, and breathing.[16]

LPIs require special attention given the risk of respiratory complications. LPIs should be monitored for increased rate and work of breathing, especially during transition. When clinically stable, skin-to-skin should be implemented to minimize infant stress, optimize respiration and oxygenation, and safeguard from hypothermia-induced apnea.[16] Parents should be educated on their LPI's risk of respiratory complications and the signs and symptoms of distress. The family also should be advised of the LPI's increased risk for asthma, respiratory infection, and rehospitalization during the first year of life.[17] Methods to avoid respiratory infections, including proper

Table 1
Late preterm development and common morbidities

Clinical Manifestation	LPI Development	Indications for Care
Respiratory		
RDS	• LPIs experience an interruption in the development and remodeling of the respiratory bronchioles and alveoli altering surfactant synthesis and secretion, and gas exchange.	• Monitor rate and work of breathing especially during transition. • Promote skin-to-skin when infant is medically stable.
TTN	• LPIs can experience ineffective clearance of fetal fluid.	• Signs of TTN can last up to 72 h.
Apnea	• LPIs have decreased ventilatory response to increased carbon dioxide levels. • LPIs have a biphasic ventilatory response to hypoxia. • LPIS have a very compliant chest wall and upper airway.	• Evaluate for other causes of apnea, ie, sepsis. • Apnea spells typically resolve at approximately 36–37 wk postmenstrual age.
Fluid, Electrolytes, Nutrition, and Gastrointestinal		
Hypoglycemia	• LPIs have immature breakdown of glycogen in the liver (glycogenolysis), adipose tissue lipolysis, hormonal dysregulation, and decreased hepatic gluconeogenesis, and ketogenesis.	• Become familiar with the most up-to-date hypoglycemia guidelines including that of the AAP, ABM, and PES, and your hospital policy. • Monitor the LPI's glucose closely for at least 24 h.
Feeding difficulties	• LPIs have immature brain development leading to low oromotor tone, immature suck-swallow reflex. • LPIs have a higher incidence of gastroesophageal reflux.	• Monitor enteral intake, growth, wet diapers, and number of stools. • Consider increasing caloric density to help optimize growth. • Provide lactation support when necessary. • Supplement with vitamin D and iron for optimal bone mineralization and brain growth and development.
Hematology		
Hyperbilirubinemia	• LPIs have increased hemoglobin breakdown resulting in an increased bilirubin load. • LPIs have increased enterohepatic circulation or gastrointestinal bilirubin reabsorption. • LPIs have decreased albumin levels.	• Promote frequent feedings. • Follow bilirubin levels. • Discharged infant should have a bilirubin level check 24–48 h after discharge.

(*continued on next page*)

Table 1
(*continued*)

Clinical Manifestation	LPI Development	Indications for Care
Neurologic		
Poor neurologic outcomes	• LPIs have immature nervous systems.	• Developmental follow-up should be considered for those infants who are very ill during hospitalization to minimize sequalae.
Other		
Thermal instability/cold stress	• LPIs have less subcutaneous fat than term infants. • LPIs have nonkeratinized thin skin. • LPIs have an immature response to temperature receptors. • LPIs have a higher surface area–to–body mass ratio. • LPIs have less brown adipose tissue.	• Provide a neutral thermal environment. • Encourage skin-to-skin in the medically stable infant. • Bathing should be postponed until the infant exhibits thermal, respiratory, and cardiovascular stability. • Educate parents on methods to prevent cold stress.

Abbreviations: AAP, American Academy of Pediatrics; ABM, Academy of Breastfeeding Medicine; LPI, late preterm infant; PES, Pediatric Endocrine Society; RDS, respiratory distress syndrome; TTN, transient tachypnea of the newborn.

hand hygiene, maintaining current immunizations, and avoiding large crowds and sick people, should be reinforced.

HYPOGLYCEMIA

Hypoglycemia affects newborn infants of all gestational ages who have not had any form of exogenous nutrition while still managing the sudden loss of maternal glucose.[17] Hypoglycemia occurs most commonly in infants with risk factors including prematurity, small for gestational age, large for gestational age, infants of diabetic mothers, maternal tocolytic therapy, genetic syndromes, and significant stressors, such as perinatal asphyxia, hypothermia, and resuscitation, and late preterm.[18–20] Preterm infants have immature breakdown of glycogen in the liver (glycogenolysis), adipose tissue lipolysis, hormonal dysregulation, decreased hepatic gluconeogenesis, and ketogenesis.[17] Usually, blood glucose concentrations among preterm infants decrease to a nadir 1 hour after birth, then rise and stabilize 3 hours after birth until metabolic pathways assume control or glucose is provided through feedings or intravenous dextrose.[17,21]

Although there is no consensus for the definition of hypoglycemia, studies have shown that a glucose concentration of less than 47 mg/dL offers the greatest predictive power.[22] In 2004, Wang and colleagues[23] showed a 15% incidence of hypoglycemia in the LPI population. When low plasma glucose levels are prolonged or recurrent, the results can be acute systemic effects and neurologic sequelae.[22] The clinical signs of hypoglycemia include an abnormal cry, poor feeding, hypothermia, diaphoresis, tremors and jitteriness, hypotonia, irritability, lethargy, seizures, cyanosis, pallor, tachypnea, apnea, and cardiac arrest.[18,22] Treatment should be based on clinical presentation and not by glucose concentration alone.[18,22]

The health care team should be aware of the most recent hypoglycemia guidelines, including the American Academy of Pediatrics (AAP), Pediatric Endocrine Society, and Academy of Breastfeeding Medicine, as well as individual hospital protocols.[18,20,24] Because LPIs are more vulnerable to low glucose concentrations, they require close monitoring for at least 24 hours.[18,22] It is also important to closely monitor LPIs' temperatures to prevent hypothermia, because cold stress can lead to worsened hypoglycemia among LPIs.[25]

NUTRITION/GASTROINTESTINAL

Feeding challenges in LPIs predispose them to longer hospital stays and hospital readmissions. LPIs have fewer awake-alert periods, which can result in decreased nutritional intake, and when combined with high energy demands, can lead to dehydration, and/or poor growth.[25] In 2004, Wang and colleagues[23] showed that 27% of all LPIs received intravenous fluid (IV) due to various clinical conditions, including poor feeding, compared with 5% of term infants.[23] Gastrointestinal immaturity is another factor that leads to feeding problems and impacts weight gain in LPIs. Preterm infants have a higher incidence of gastroesophageal reflux (GER) due to transient relaxation of the lower esophageal sphincter.[26] GER can have a cascading effect, leading to dehydration and hypernatremia in the initial weeks after birth.[13]

Immature brain development, including low oromotor tone, is another reason LPIs have feeding challenges, lack adequate oral intake, and are predisposed to dehydration, poor growth, and hyperbilirubinemia.[17] During the final weeks of gestation, oral motor skills become more coordinated, and movements become smoother, but LPIs miss this crucial period of development.[27] Additionally, LPIs have immature suck-swallow reflexes that can lead to difficulties with latching during breastfeeding and inadequate intake during bottle feeding.[25]

Management of LPIs should include educating parents on infants' sleep-wake cycles, feeding cues, and promoting postural stability while feeding.[25] Postural stability, which means ensuring hips are flexed and head and neck are in alignment with the trunk, improves feeding success in the LPI.[27] The LPI's immature brain development is often overlooked because LPIs are considered stable when compared with their extremely premature counterparts. However, the caregiver must pay special attention to provide safe and effective oral feedings. Close monitoring of adequate enteral intake in the early neonatal period is of utmost importance, and if the mother is breastfeeding, lactation support is critical because of the increased risk of difficulty in establishing effective breastfeeding.[22] If growth is not adequately maintained, calorie fortification should be considered.[22] LPIs also should be supplemented with vitamin D, for bone mineralization, and iron, which are essential for the growth and development of the brain and nervous system.[22]

THERMAL INSTABILITY/COLD STRESS

LPIs are at increased risk of thermal instability, particularly cold stress, due to their physiologic and metabolic immaturity. An understanding of the LPI's limitations can minimize morbidity and mortality. Term infants experiencing cold stress use several mechanisms to conserve and generate body heat. After the activation of temperature-specific receptors, term infants constrict their peripheral blood vessels, increase muscle flexion and activity, and metabolize brown adipose tissue (BAT), also known as nonshivering thermogenesis (NST).[28] These processes allow the term infant to maintain blood and heat in the core of the body, decrease the surface area available for heat loss, and generate heat and energy through muscle movement and fat breakdown. LPIs are more likely to experience thermal instability than the term infant because of their deficiency in subcutaneous fat, nonkeratinized thin skin, immature response to temperature receptors, high surface area–to–body mass ratio, and deficiency in BAT.[13,28,29]

NST through BAT metabolism is the major mechanism of heat production in infants. BAT cells begin to differentiate at approximately 25 to 26 weeks' gestation, and brown adipocytes can be seen at approximately 29 weeks and continue to increase until a few weeks after birth.[30] In the term infant, BAT accounts for 1% of the infant's body weight and can increase heat production by 100% or more above basal level.[13,28] In response to cold stress, norepinephrine stimulates the nerve endings on the brown fat resulting in metabolization and heat production. Blood is warmed as it passes through the various areas of BAT metabolization and, subsequently, warms the body. NST is limited in LPIs due to insufficient BAT mass.[13]

Cold stress can have deleterious effects on the LPI. In the setting of cold stress, there is a release of norepinephrine, which causes various systemic effects, each of which can increase infant morbidity and mortality. Norepinephrine release in LPIs increases their metabolic rate, oxygen consumption, and glucose utilization. To maintain an increased metabolic rate, the infant must consume more oxygen. Higher oxygen consumption can lead to hypoxemia, and, subsequently, decreased oxygen delivery to the tissues, or hypoxia. Higher metabolic rates also require higher glucose utilization, which can lead to hypoglycemia. In a population that already has a higher risk of respiratory distress and hypoglycemia, cold stress can exacerbate these conditions and increase their risk of morbidity and mortality.

Several tactics can be implemented to minimize heat loss and avoid cold stress. The provision of a neutral thermal environment is ideal for the LPI.[28] Providers and caretakers must be aware that environments that may be comfortable for an adult may require increased metabolic efforts to maintain a normal temperature in the infant. Skin-to-skin in the stable LPI should be encouraged. Most infants are able to maintain their temperature during skin-to-skin, especially if the infant is wearing a hat and a blanket.[16,28] Bathing should be postponed until the infant exhibits thermal, respiratory, and cardiovascular stability. Consider a partial rather than a full body bath, dry infant immediately after bathing, and cover the infant's head with a dry hat. Most importantly, the family should be educated on methods of heat loss (**Table 2**) and taught techniques to prevent cold stress.

HYPERBILIRUBINEMIA

Hyperbilirubinemia is the most common reason for readmission among LPIs.[31,32] Sixty percent of term infants and almost all preterm infants develop hyperbilirubinemia.[33] LPIs are 2.4 times more likely to develop hyperbilirubinemia than term infants, and it lasts longer and is more pronounced in LPIs compared with term infants.[17,34] In healthy term infants, bilirubin levels peak at 5 to 7 mg/dL at approximately 3 to 5 days of life and decline by 7 to 10 days.[33] In preterm infants, total serum bilirubin (TSB) levels peak at 10 to 12 mg/dL by the fifth day of life.[33] Infants who are breastfed have higher bilirubin levels than bottle-fed infants.[34]

Hyperbilirubinemia occurs as a result of increased bilirubin production, decreased metabolism and elimination, or a combination of the two.[13] Newborns have a higher volume of red blood cells (RBCs) per kilogram and a higher proportion of RBCs with a shorter lifespan, yielding a source for greater bilirubin production.[13,33] The lifespan

Table 2
Methods of heat loss

Method	Definition	Example
Conduction	The transfer of heat from the body surface to an object in contact with the body.	That is, heat loss to a cold scale or unwarmed mattress.
Convection	The loss of heat molecules through the skin or mucous membranes into the surrounding air. It can occur through the skin and/or the respiratory tract.	That is, heat loss from an intubated patient to a cool ventilator circuit or a naked infant to a cool room.
Evaporation	The loss of heat as moisture on the skin vaporizes. This process is always accompanied by a cooling effect.	That is, heat loss in the delivery room immediately after birth (amniotic fluid) or after a bath.
Radiation	The transfer of heat between solid surfaces that are not in direct contact with each other.	That is, loss to a cold window or incubator wall.

of RBCs in term newborns is 80 to 100 days, whereas the RBC lifespan in preterm infants is 60 to 80 days, predisposing the preterm infant to greater breakdown of hemoglobin and an increased bilirubin load.[33] LPIs have decreased activity of the UGT gene that is required by the liver enzyme glucuronyl transferase to conjugate indirect bilirubin to direct bilirubin, a water-soluble, excretable form of bilirubin, leading to an increased indirect bilirubin load.[13,33]

LPIs have immature gastrointestinal function and feeding difficulties that predispose them to increased enterohepatic circulation, or gastrointestinal bilirubin reabsorption.[17] These factors contribute to hyperbilirubinemia, decreased stool frequency, and dehydration.[17] Additionally, newborns have decreased levels of albumin compared with older infants and adults, and the levels are even lower in preterm and LPIs.[33] Albumin carries bilirubin to the liver to be conjugated, and decreased albumin means there are fewer binding sites for bilirubin, resulting in an increased amount of free bilirubin, which causes neurotoxicity in infants.[33,35]

According to AAP guidelines, to prevent adverse outcomes, clinicians should promote frequent and successful breastfeeding.[33,36] Facilities should have protocols in place to identify infants at risk for hyperbilirubinemia, and clinicians should measure a bilirubin level on jaundiced infants in the first 24 hours, and treat infants when appropriate.[36] It is important, as well, to provide verbal and written information to parents on neonatal hyperbilirubinemia.[36]

Phototherapy is the most widely used therapeutic modality in infants with hyperbilirubinemia, followed by exchange transfusion, and intravenous immune globulin.[37] Twenty-five percent of LPIs will require phototherapy.[23] The goal of treatment is to prevent severe neonatal hyperbilirubinemia, acute bilirubin encephalopathy, and ultimately, kernicterus.[36] The signs of acute bilirubin encephalopathy include hypertonia, arching, retrocollis, opisthotonos, fever, and a high-pitched cry.[36] The possible causes of hyperbilirubinemia should be explored in infants receiving phototherapy or whose TSB levels are rising rapidly.[36] Conditions that can complicate and prolong hyperbilirubinemia include Rh isoimmunization, ABO incompatibility, and genetic disorders, such as glucose-6-phosphate dehydrogenase deficiency.[32]

NEUROLOGIC DEVELOPMENT

When compared with term infants, preterm infants have an immature central nervous system. The preterm infant's brain size is approximately two-thirds the size of a full-term infant's brain.[6,22] The preterm brain has fewer sulci and gyri, and the weight of the brain at 34 weeks is 65% of that of a term infant.[6,22] It is between 34 and 40 weeks' gestational age that cortical volume increases by 50%, and 25% of cerebellar development takes place.[38,39] These factors place preterm infants at an increased risk for altered brain development, which may influence long-term neurodevelopmental outcomes.[22,40]

LPIs have a threefold increased risk of cerebral palsy compared with term infants.[6] In 2016, Prachi and colleagues[41] concluded that children born in the late preterm period demonstrate poorer performance on tests of early school readiness, spatial abilities, and verbal reasoning in early childhood, poorer educational achievement at age 5, and poorer school performance at age 7. In 2015, Dusing and Tripathi[40] concluded LPIs are at risk of having reduced long-term neurodevelopmental outcomes, with cognition being at the highest risk and persisting the longest. The review by Dusing and Tripathi[40] also concluded there is an increased risk of neurodevelopmental delay in LPIs up to 18 years of age when compared with infants born at term. LPIs account for 72% of all preterm births, and even the smallest increases in adverse outcomes could translate to a large public health burden.[42]

MORBIDITY

LPIs are often viewed as functionally mature when, indeed, they are not. This population was previously referred to as "near term," erroneously giving the connotation that nothing more than routine surveillance was required. However, "near term" was changed to "late preterm" to channel the susceptibility of LPIs. An LPI birth is complicated by the arrest in growth and development of vital systems,[6] and is associated with significant short-term and long-term morbidities. In fact, LPIs have a sixfold to sevenfold greater morbidity rate than term infants, a rate that rises with other neonatal morbidity risk factors.[43,44]

Increased neonatal morbidities have been associated with maternal prenatal complications. Conditions, including chorioamnionitis, premature rupture of membranes, hypertension, preeclampsia, diabetes, and maternal smoking, are common maternal complications seen with LPI births.[6] The neonatal complication of intrauterine growth restriction is also more common in the LPI. Although most LPIs will have a benign neonatal course, LPIs continue to have a higher risk of morbidity than the term infant. Morbidities, including respiratory problems requiring mechanical ventilation, apnea, sepsis, feeding problems, jaundice, hypoglycemia, temperature instability, and intraventricular hemorrhage, occur more frequently in the LPI population.[43,44] Higher rates of emergency department visits for apnea/apparent life-threatening events, feeding problems, dehydration, jaundice, and sepsis have also been reported.[44]

MORTALITY

Although the relative risk of mortality in the LPI compared with the term infant is small, the mortality rate is 4 times higher in the LPI.[5] In 2016, Bulut and colleagues[2] reported the number one cause of death in the LPI was respiratory distress. This same study also reported a higher rate of death from respiratory distress, pneumonia, perinatal asphyxia, and sepsis in the LPI compared with the term infant.[2] Mortality was also increased with elective Cesarean deliveries, placental complications, newborn bacterial sepsis, antepartum hemorrhage, and hypertensive disorders.[6] Several studies have reported an increased risk of neonatal death with decreasing gestational age.[2,45] In a population of LPIs and term infants, a mortality rate as high as 8.2 per 1000 live births was reported at 34 weeks' gestation compared with 0.5 per 1000 live births for term infants born at 40 weeks' gestation.[45]

COST OF CARE

The cost of care for LPIs is higher than that of the term infant and can be attributed to many factors. The 2006 Institute of Medicine report *Preterm births: Causes, Consequences and Prevention* estimated the total annual cost of preterm births to be more than $26 billion per year, attributing nearly two-thirds of the cost to medical care.[46] Although this figure was inclusive of all preterm infants less than 37 weeks' gestational age, several studies have attempted to capture the cost of the LPI.[4,47,48] To gather a complete picture of the total cost of the LPI, it is necessary to include antepartum management, delivery cost, cost of care during the neonatal period, and long-term needs, including medical, educational, and social services. Although it may not be easily quantified, the impact of preterm birth on family psychological health and stress levels also should be considered.

Gestational age and cost of care have an inverse relationship. In 2010, Loftin and colleagues[8] reported the average cost for a single infant born at 34, 35, and 36 weeks' gestation was estimated to be $7200, $4200, and $2600, respectively.[8] When the total number of births was annualized, the cost translated to $41.4 million, $41.1 million, and $42.8 million at 34, 35, and 36 weeks, respectively.

LPIs have higher rates of morbidity immediately after birth and higher readmission rates during infancy and their first year of life.[4,48] It has been reported that LPIs between 34 0/7 and 34 6/7 weeks' gestation have as high as a ninefold increased risk of long-term morbidity and continual use of health care resources.[8] LPIs often have a longer length of hospital stay after birth. In a retrospective study of commercially insured infants in the United States, LPIs averaged 8.8 days in the hospital with an average cost of $26,054 versus 2.2 hospital days and an average cost of $2061 for term infants.[4] In 2009, McLaurin and colleagues[4] reported hospital readmission rates to be 2 to 3 times greater for LPIs compared with term infants. During the first year after discharge, medical cost was reported as much as 3 times higher in LPIs compared with term infants.[43] This was echoed in a study of Arkansas Medicaid claims data, which reported that LPIs had higher outpatient and inpatient Medicaid expenses during the first year compared with the term infant.[48]

DISCHARGE PLANNING/FOLLOW-UP

There is a high number of readmissions in the LPI population, and this population is particularly at risk for readmission related to hyperbilirubinemia, apparent life-threatening events or apnea, feeding problems, possible sepsis, hypothermia, and respiratory problems.[49] LPIs warrant specific medical monitoring and nutritional practices to optimize their growth and positive outcomes.[22] Careful discharge planning for the LPI may help prevent hospital readmissions and lead to positive long-term outcomes (**Box 1**).

Box 1
Discharge planning for the late preterm infant

- Infants must have a carefully documented assessment of gestational age.
- Before discharge, infants must demonstrate an established feeding pattern with adequate volumes and calories to promote growth and prevent dehydration.
- Infants must be able to maintain temperatures of 36.5 to 37.4° Celsius (97.7–99.3°F) in an open crib without excessive clothing.
- If apnea of prematurity is identified as a diagnosis, the infant must have a documented period free of apnea based on the institution's policy.
- Perform a systematic assessment on all infants before discharge for the risk of severe hyperbilirubinemia.
- Provide parents with written and verbal information about newborn jaundice.
- Provide appropriate hyperbilirubinemia follow-up based on the time of discharge and the risk assessment.
- A primary care provider must be identified before discharge, and the first appointment must be scheduled within 24 to 48 hours after discharge.
- A car seat safety study must be completed by a trained professional with documentation the infant passed.
- Newborn metabolic screenings have been submitted according to requirements mandated by each state.
- The infant has received the first Hepatitis B vaccine, or arrangements have been made for the infant to get the vaccine in the pediatrician's office.
- Late preterm infants (LPIs) of less than 36 weeks' gestational age should be considered at risk for infection and managed according to current guidelines for prevention of group B streptococcal infection.
- Educate parents on RSV (respiratory syncytial virus), most common from fall to spring, RSV prophylaxis, and preventing the spread of RSV.
- Educate parents on avoiding exposure of infant to people with active upper respiratory tract infections or other viral infections.
- Educate parents on avoiding exposure of infant to second-hand and third-hand smoke.
- To help prevent sudden infant death syndrome, educate parents on infants sleeping alone and on their backs with no additional bedding.
- LPIs are generally not scheduled for developmental follow-up; however, developmental surveillance is important given the risk of adverse long-term developmental outcomes in this population.

SUMMARY

Most LPIs will fare well, however, this population is met with challenges unique to this age group. They often experience morbidities that can prolong hospital stays and lead to hospital readmissions, often related to feeding problems, dehydration, hypothermia, jaundice, and apparent life-threatening events. The LPI population also experiences mortality rates 4 times higher than the rates for term infants.[5] With diligent surveillance by the health care team and caregivers, challenges in the LPI population can be addressed before they become life-threatening or lead to long-term adverse outcomes that could translate to a large public health burden.

REFERENCES

1. Jacob J, Lehne M, Mischker A, et al. Cost effects of preterm birth: a comparison of health care costs associated with early preterm, late preterm, and full-term birth in the first 3 years after birth. Eur J Health Econ 2017;18(8):1041–6. Available at: https://search.proquest.com/docview/1939197821.
2. Bulut C, Gürsoy T, Ovalı F. Short-term outcomes and mortality of late preterm infants. Balkan Med J 2016;33(2):198–203. Available at: http://www.ncbi.nlm.nih.gov/pubmed/27403390.
3. Shapiro-Mendoza CK, Tomashek KM, Kotelchuck M, et al. Effect of late-preterm birth and maternal medical conditions on newborn morbidity risk. Pediatrics 2008;121(2):223.
4. McLaurin KK, Hall CB, Jackson EA, et al. Persistence of morbidity and cost differences between late-preterm and term infants during the first year of life. Pediatrics 2009;123(2):653–9. Available at: http://pediatrics.aappublications.org/cgi/content/abstract/123/2/653.
5. The Consortium on Safe Labor. Respiratory morbidity in late preterm births. JAMA 2010;304(4):419–25.
6. Kugelman A, Colin AA. Late preterm infants: near term but still in a critical developmental time period. Pediatrics 2013;132(4):741–51. Available at: http://www.ncbi.nlm.nih.gov/pubmed/24062372.
7. Bassil K, Shah P, Shah V, et al. Impact of late preterm and early term infants on Canadian neonatal intensive care units. Am J Perinatol 2014;31(4):269–78. Available at: http://www.thieme-connect.de/DOI/DOI?10.1055/s-0033-1347364.
8. Loftin RW, Habli M, Snyder CC, et al. Late preterm birth. Rev Obstet Gynecol 2010;3(1):10. Available at: http://www.ncbi.nlm.nih.gov/pubmed/20508778.
9. Chung EK, Gable EK, Golden WK, et al. Current scope of practice for newborn care in non-intensive hospital settings. Hosp Pediatr 2017;7(8):471–82.
10. Kallapur SG, Jobe AH. Lung development and maturation. In: Martin R, Fanaroff A, Walsh M, editors. Fanaroff and Martin's neonatal-perinatal medicine. 10th edition. Saunders; 2015. p. 1042–59. Available at: https://www.clinicalkey.es/playcontent/3-s2.0-B9781455756179000701.
11. Wert SE. Normal and abnormal structural development of the lung. In: Polin RA, Abman SH, Rowitch DH, et al, editors. Fetal and neonatal physiology. 5th edition. Elsevier; 2017. p. 641.e3. Available at: https://www.clinicalkey.es/playcontent/3-s2.0-B9780323352147000615.
12. Ramachandrappa A, Jain L. The late preterm infant. In: Martin R, Fanaroff A, Walsh M, editors. Fanaroff and Martin's neonatal-perinatal medicine: diseases of the fetus and infant. 10th edition. Saunders; 2015. p. 577–91.
13. Raju TNK. Developmental physiology of late and moderate prematurity. Semin Fetal Neonatal Med 2012;17(3):126. Available at: http://www.sciencedirect.com/science/article/pii/S1744165X1200011X.
14. Laptook AR. Neurologic and metabolic issues in moderately preterm, late preterm, and early term infants. Clin Perinatol 2013;40(4):723–38. Available at: http://www.ncbi.nlm.nih.gov/pubmed/24182958.
15. Teune MJ, Bakhuizen S, Gyamfi Bannerman C, et al. A systematic review of severe morbidity in infants born late preterm. Am J Obstet Gynecol 2011;205(4):374.e1-e9. Available at: http://www.sciencedirect.com/science/article/pii/S0002937811009161.

16. Phillips RM, Goldstein M, Hougland K, et al. Multidisciplinary guidelines for the care of late preterm infants. J Perinatol 2013;33(S2):S5. Available at: http://www.ncbi.nlm.nih.gov/pubmed/23803627.
17. Engle WA, Tomashek KM, Wallman C, Committee on Fetus and Newborn. "Late-preterm" infants: a population at risk. Pediatrics 2007;120(6):1390–401. Available at: http://aappolicy.aappublications.org/cgi/content/abstract/pediatrics;120/6/1390.
18. Adamkin DH. Postnatal glucose homeostasis in late-preterm and term infants. Pediatrics 2011;127(3):575–9. Available at: http://www.ncbi.nlm.nih.gov/pubmed/21357346.
19. Askin DF. Complications in the transition from fetal to neonatal life. J Obstet Gynecol Neonatal Nurs 2002;31(3):318–27. Available at: http://onlinelibrary.wiley.com/doi/10.1111/j.1552-6909.2002.tb00054.x/abstract.
20. Thornton PS, Stanley CA, De Leon DD, et al. Recommendations from the Pediatric Endocrine Society for evaluation and management of persistent hypoglycemia in neonates, infants, and children. J Pediatr 2015;167(2):238–45. Available at: https://www.sciencedirect.com/science/article/pii/S0022347615003583.
21. Ward Platt M, Deshpande S. Metabolic adaptation at birth. Semin Fetal Neonatal Med 2005;10(4):341–50. Available at: http://www.sciencedirect.com/science/article/pii/S1744165X05000181.
22. Polin RA, Yoder MC. Workbook in practical neonatology. Elsevier Health Sciences; 2014. Available at: http://lib.myilibrary.com?ID=755774.
23. Wang ML, Dorer DJ, Fleming MP, et al. Clinical outcomes of near-term infants. Pediatrics 2004;114(2):372–6. Available at: http://pediatrics.aappublications.org/cgi/content/abstract/114/2/372.
24. Wight N, Marinelli KA. ABM clinical protocol #1: guidelines for blood glucose monitoring and treatment of hypoglycemia in term and late-preterm neonates, revised 2014. Breastfeed Med 2014;9(4):173–9. Available at: http://www.liebertonline.com/doi/abs/10.1089/bfm.2014.9986.
25. Cleaveland K. Feeding challenges in the late preterm infant. Neonatal Netw 2010;29(1):37–41. Available at: http://www.ncbi.nlm.nih.gov/pubmed/20085875.
26. Martin R, Hibbs A. Gastroesophageal reflux in premature infants. UpToDate; 2017.
27. Ludwig SM. Oral feeding and the late preterm infant. Newborn Infant Nurs Rev 2007;7(2):72–5. Available at: http://www.sciencedirect.com/science/article/pii/S1527336907000463.
28. Blackburn S. Maternal, fetal, & neonatal physiology. 4th edition. Saint Louis (MO): Saunders; 2012. p. 664–71. Available at: http://replace-me/ebraryid=11067435.
29. Karlsen K. The stable program. 6th edition. Salt Lake City (UT): 2013. p. 64–83.
30. Hamilton BE, Martin JA, Osterman MJK, et al. Births: Provisional data for 2017. Vital Statistics Rapid Release; no 4. Hyattsville (MD): National Center for Health Statistics; 2018. p. 002. Available at: https://www.cdc.gov/nchs/data/vsrr/report004.pdf.
31. Raju TNK. The problem of late-preterm (near-term) births: a workshop summary. Pediatr Res 2006;60(6):775–6. Available at: http://www.ncbi.nlm.nih.gov/pubmed/17065577.
32. U.S. National Library of Medicine. Glucose-6-phosphate dehydrogenase deficiency. 2017. Available at: https://ghr.nlm.nih.gov/condition/glucose-6-phosphate-dehydrogenase-deficiency#definition. Accessed September 25, 2017.

33. Watson RL. Hyperbilirubinemia. Crit Care Nurs Clin North Am 2009;21(1):97–120. Available at: http://www.sciencedirect.com/science/article/pii/S0899588508000956.
34. Martin R, Fanaroff A, Walsh M. Fanaroff and Martin's neonatal-perinatal medicine. 9th edition. Philadelphia: Elsevier Health Sciences; 2011. p. 1496. Available at: http://www.r2library.com/resource/title/9780323065450.
35. Amin SB, Lamola AA. Newborn jaundice technologies: unbound bilirubin and bilirubin binding capacity in neonates. Semin Perinatol 2011;35(3):134–40. Available at: http://www.sciencedirect.com/science/article/pii/S014600051100036X.
36. Subcommittee on Hyperbilirubinemia. Management of hyperbilirubinemia in the newborn infant 35 or more weeks of gestation. Pediatrics 2004;114(1): 297–316. Available at: http://aappolicy.aappublications.org/cgi/content/abstract/pediatrics;114/1/297.
37. Hansen T. Neonatal jaundice. Medscape; 2016. Available at: https://emedicine.medscape.com/article/974786-overview?pa=8BkebdrflK5ictVYRyFRJm4AkRsXxZeJ8g5oM9A7wBQVazSqkaLX9ccc03qbRC82HuhjYMIXEPDr2F0EKwK%2BFOejCO3Rk4DWsD37DrSZWvU%3D.
38. Kapellou O, Counsell SJ, Kennea N, et al. Abnormal cortical development after premature birth shown by altered allometric scaling of brain growth. PLoS Med 2006;3(8):e265. Available at: http://www.ncbi.nlm.nih.gov/pubmed/16866579.
39. Kinney HC. The near-term (late preterm) human brain and risk for periventricular leukomalacia: a review. Semin Perinatol 2006;30(2):81–8. Available at: http://www.sciencedirect.com/science/article/pii/S0146000506000437.
40. Dusing S, Tripathi T. Long-term neurodevelopmental outcomes of infants born late preterm: a systematic review. Res Rep Neonatol 2015;2015:91–111. Available at: https://doaj.org/article/15cd250d054f418dbf1a435b25c5d9fe.
41. Prachi S, Kaciroti N, Richards B, et al. Developmental outcomes of late preterm infants from infancy to kindergarten. Pediatrics 2016;138(2):1. Available at: https://search.proquest.com/docview/1812901617.
42. Cheong JL, Doyle LW, Burnett AC, et al. Association between moderate and late preterm birth and neurodevelopment and social-emotional development at age 2 years. JAMA Pediatr 2017;171(4):e164805.
43. Barfield W, Lee K. Late preterm infants. In: Weisman L, Kim M, editors. UpToDate. Waltham (MA): UpToDate; 2017. Available at: http://www.uptodate.com/contents/late-preterm-infants. Accessed August 9, 2017.
44. Chang HJ. Long-term cognition, achievement, socioemotional, and behavioral development of healthy late-preterm infants. JAMA 2010;304(7):727. Available at: https://search.proquest.com/docview/748908361.
45. Young PC, Glasgow TS, Li X, et al. Mortality of late-preterm (near-term) newborns in Utah. Pediatrics 2007;119(3):e665. Available at: http://pediatrics.aappublications.org/cgi/content/abstract/119/3/e659.
46. Committee on Understanding Premature Birth and Assuring Healthy Outcomes. Preterm birth: causes, consequences, and prevention. Washington, DC: National Academies Press; 2006. Available at: http://lib.myilibrary.com?ID=84458.
47. Berard A, Le Tiec M, De Vera MA, et al. Study of the costs and morbidities of late-preterm birth. Arch Dis Child Fetal Neonatal Ed 2012;97(5):f334.
48. Bird TM, Bronstein JM, Hall RW, et al. Late preterm infants: birth outcomes and health care utilization in the first year. Pediatrics 2010;126(2):e319. Available at: http://www.ncbi.nlm.nih.gov/pubmed/20603259.
49. Whyte R. Safe discharge of the late preterm infant. Paediatr Child Health 2010; 15(10):655. Available at: http://www.ncbi.nlm.nih.gov/pubmed/22131865.

Increased Nursing Participation in Multidisciplinary Rounds to Enhance Communication, Patient Safety, and Parent Satisfaction

Karen Dittman, MSN, CRNP, NNP-BC*, Stephanie Hughes, RN, BSN

KEYWORDS

- Multidisciplinary rounds • ICU • Nursing role • Patient safety • Communication
- Satisfaction

KEY POINTS

- Bedside nurses have unique and vital information to contribute to the assessment and care of neonatal ICU (NICU) patients.
- Active nursing participation in multidisciplinary patient rounds increases communication between members of the medical team, with the goal of improving patient safety and patient/parent satisfaction.
- Nursing staff education and support are vital for the successful transition to NICU multidisciplinary rounds.
- Developing a rounding script as a tool for nurses during multidisciplinary rounding and shift report contributed to project success.

BACKGROUND

Effective communication among health care team members is a mainstay of patient safety, especially in a neonatal ICU (NICU), where errors can lead to serious harm. These errors have the potential to be life threatening with long-term consequences. In addition, ineffective communication with families of hospitalized children can lead to decreased satisfaction and levels of inherent trust of the health care team. To improve medical team communication and parent satisfaction, the nursing staff at the Johns Hopkins Children's Center's NICU spearheaded an initiative to create an

Disclosure: The authors have nothing to disclose.
Neonatal Intensive Care Unit, The Johns Hopkins Hospital, Charlotte R. Bloomberg Children's Center, 1800 Orleans Street, Baltimore, MD 21287, USA
* Corresponding author.
E-mail address: kdittma2@jhmi.edu

Crit Care Nurs Clin N Am 30 (2018) 445–455
https://doi.org/10.1016/j.cnc.2018.07.002 ccnursing.theclinics.com
0899-5885/18/

enhanced nursing role for multidisciplinary patient rounds. This required a change in practice for nursing staff, medical providers, and other members of the multidisciplinary team. Successful implementation of the changeover involved education of the nursing staff and other team members, coordination of NICU workflows, and development of a rounding script for nurses to be used as an outline for patient presentations on rounds as well as a handoff tool for shift-to-shift bedside reports.

The NICU at the Johns Hopkins Children's Center is a 45-bed tertiary-care unit located within an academic medical center that delivers care to many premature and critically ill infants in the geographic region. Most of the neonates have highly complex medical and surgical conditions, and the NICU and parents rely heavily on the bedside nurse to be expert caregivers, advocates, and gatekeepers for their assigned patients. Family members also depend on the nursing staff to act as a care guide given the strange milieu of the NICU and to assist them in deciphering a vast array of unfamiliar information and terminology. Members of the NICU nursing staff witnessed an opportunity to improve communication, patient safety, and family satisfaction by more fully utilizing the intimate and unique knowledge possessed by the bedside nurse. To achieve this goal, modification of the manner in which daily rounds were conducted in the NICU needed to be overhauled and modified.

The impetus for the change to increase nursing participation on rounds and ultimately develop truly multidisciplinary rounds was conceived by the patient satisfaction committee within the NICU. Parents had periodically indicated in satisfaction surveys that vague and unclear communication was a concern, with the information they received from nursing staff sometimes differing from information they received from other members of the medical team. Parents were often distressed when they received conflicting information regarding plans of care or updates on test results, which led to increased parental stress and anxiety as well as decreased levels of parent satisfaction. This stress and anxiety can transform and evolve into distrust of the health care team. A systematic review of the impact of pediatric critical illness on families conducted by Shudy and colleagues[1] identified communication difficulties with staff to be a stressor for families and that staff communication and actions became a more significant stressor over time. Given the protracted hospital stays of critically ill newborns, trust in the medical team, most importantly the bedside nurse with whom they have the most connection, is important for the emotional well-being of family members. Parents often view the NICU nurses as a surrogate parent to their infant and developed attachments to individual nurses. When information and updates parents received from the assigned nurse slightly or significantly differed from the information received from other members of the medical team, parental anxiety and stress were exponentially elevated. Ann Wills, the mother of a NICU patient, in a commentary for *Pediatric Nursing*, describes "how confusing it was to hear different things from different team members of the same team and also to hear conflicting information between differing teams."[2] The patient satisfaction committee members understood that clear and accurate communication between families and members of the health care team was vital to the establishment of a healthy partnership between the 2 parties.

Additional discussion within the committee focused on abundant research that optimal communication among health care team members results in improved patient safety and quality outcome indicators. Communication failures within health care systems are one of the leading causes of inadvertent patient harm, and having all team members on the same page has been shown to decrease adverse events.[3] Given the complex nature of care within the NICU, strategies to increase accurate and timely communication had already been implemented. The NICU team already used huddles to enhance communication and safety within the unit. The main morning huddle occurred before rounds and included the nurse manager, charge nurses, discharge coordinator, nurse practitioners, attending neonatologists from each rounding team, neonatal fellow of the day, member of the transport team, lead respiratory therapist, and social worker among others. This huddle provided an opportunity for the planning and coordination by all team members regarding anticipated deliveries, discharges, transfers, scheduled and unscheduled surgeries, and intrahospital diagnostic testing. It also identified potential hot spots within the NICU to enhance awareness among staff members. A hot spot, for example, could be a cluster of medically unstable neonates. An abbreviated version of the huddle was conducted in the evening to coordinate overnight concerns. Nurses and respiratory therapists also participated in hallway huddles on each shift to identify patients and situations that could require extra attention and responsiveness.

A few committee members had previously worked in other patient care units where nurses had a more significant role during rounds and shared collective thoughts that nurse-led rounds might improve communication within the unit, thereby improving patient safety as well as parent satisfaction. Research has also shown greater job satisfaction for nurses when they sense they are an integral part of the team.[4,5] On further discussion, a core group of the committee met with NICU nursing leadership to discuss the feasibility of such a change in unit practice, which was met with approval and support. The core group also met with the NICU medical director to discuss the proposal, and, with their input, the decision was made to proceed with the development of a more multidisciplinary approach to unit rounding.

The NICU care delivery model consists of 2 medical teams, each led by an attending neonatologist, with 1 team composed of residents and a fellow, known as the Doc team, and the other team composed of neonatal nurse practitioners (NNPs), known as the NNP team. Patient acuity is essentially equal for both teams. The 45-bed unit is arranged in a pattern of 4 hallways with private patient rooms along both sides of each hallway. Patients from each team are distributed more or less evenly among the hallways. Daily patient rounds take place midmorning with both teams rounding concurrently. Rounds are conducted at the bedside of each neonate. From a historical perspective, patient information and daily updates were presented by the assigned resident or nurse practitioner during rounds. As such, a system-based plan of care was then developed under the guidance of the neonatologist. Other personnel participating on rounds could include the bedside nurse, respiratory therapist, nutritionist, clinical pharmacist, and rounding nurse. The size of the team ranged between 6 and 10 participants, with 3 to 4 mobile computer stations accompanying each team for data and note entry. Parents of patients were also welcomed and encouraged to attend rounds. Nurses were able to contribute to the discussion but did not formally present the patient. Nursing presence was encouraged but given individual patient care responsibilities it was not always feasible from a workload perspective. Due to the high acuity of the unit, rounds often were interrupted by an admission or other urgent patient need, or the information presented was fragmented or incomplete if the bedside nurse and respiratory therapist were unable to be present and contribute vital data. This lead to incomplete communication, with the bedside nurse unaware of changes to the medical plan or new orders written during rounds which could delay patient care. In addition, she may need to locate and clarify any changes with the medical provider while rounds were proceeding on other patients, thus slowing down rounds. With the integration of multidisciplinary rounding into the care delivery system, the bedside nurse played a central role in rounds, ensuring timely and accurate conveyance of patient information and the development of an appropriate daily plan of care.

METHODS

The first step to using this initiative was for members of the committee to observe other units where nursing participation was already integrated into the care delivery model. Committee members visited the pediatric ICU (PICU) within the Johns Hopkins Hospital Children's Center, another large NICU in the geographic region, and a smaller NICU in Baltimore city to observe rounds. In the smaller NICU, rounds at the bedside included the medical providers, pharmacist, nutritionist, bedside nurse (if available), and charge nurse. On this unit, the presentation of patient data was by a medical provider and used a similar systems-based approach. The bedside nurse listened but did not contribute unless asked a direct question or had essential information to share. It was observed that the nurse was often not able to be present while rounds were conducted due to other patient care duties. The committee members concluded this visit with the impressions that participation of the nurse was ancillary and reflective of suboptimal team integration. Such an arrangement did not meet the objective for increased nursing participation.

In the PICU within the Johns Hopkins Children's Center and in another large NICU within the Baltimore metropolitan region, the nursing role was more central to the rounding process. The assigned nurse presented the entirety of the patient information, including the name, age, diagnosis, weight change, interval history, vital signs, laboratory results, current lines, wounds and drains, infusions and medications, and physical assessment. The assigned medical provider, whether resident or nurse practitioner, followed with an assessment and the development of the daily plan under the direction of the attending physician was formulated. All team members, as well as parents, were encouraged to participate in the process. The nurses who presented on rounds used printed paper scripts completed by the off-going night shift nurse. These scripts were used to give the shift-to-shift report in addition to facilitating rounds. Day shift nurses updated the scripts after rounds and throughout the shift and again used the scripts to give report to the oncoming night shift nurse. The committee had several members who had previously worked in the PICU and were instrumental in advocating this style of daily rounding.

After the unit visits were completed, all patient satisfaction committee members reviewed *A Foundation for Patient Safety: Phase I Implementation of Interdisciplinary Bedside Rounds in the Pediatric Intensive Care Unit*, by Licata and colleagues,[6] which describes the implementation of a similar effort in another unit. The committee developed a rough outline for rounding that nurses used as a rounding script. The new format not only allowed or encouraged the participation of nurses during rounds but also made their participation central to the process. With the input of the medical director, a multidisciplinary approach was developed with the nurse central to the process but with other team members presenting sections as well (refer to **Box 1** for the program mission).

Pivotal to the success of increased nursing participation on rounds was the development and utilization of the rounding script to aid nurses in the orderly presentation of pertinent data. With the assistance of the NICU medical director, a sequence for presenting on rounds was developed that synced with information contained in the electronic medical record, which auto-populates into the daily note written by the medical team. The rounding script was a 4-page document, printed on card stock, and updated nightly by the assigned overnight nurse. The script then was used by the assigned day shift nurse to present the patient on rounds. It also was used by the nurses to give the shift-to-shift report, thus replacing the individual report sheets. The rounding script went through many revisions during development to increase

Box 1
Program mission

- To improve patient safety by improving communication
- To encourage collaboration between nurses, respiratory therapists, nutritionists, pharmacists, providers, and family members
- To ensure shared decision making between all providers and family members
- To reduce length of stay and readmissions
- To improve patient satisfaction
- To elevate the bedside nurse's role as a leader with the presentation of key patient information
- To increase attention to patient and family-centered care

utility and optimize user-friendly status. Changes to the script were made to include new initiatives instituted within the NICU. For example, the rounding script was modified to contain a section on kangaroo care (KC), including eligibility for KC and documenting when KC was last done. This was a concurrent initiative in the NICU with the goal of increasing the rate of participation in KC. In addition to rounding material, the script contained information the nurses needed to share during patient handoff at shift change, such as medication and feeding times, that did not need to be presented during rounds. Shaded headers on the rounding script distinguished between each type of information and also indicated the individual responsible for presenting each section during rounds. A rounding script is shown in Appendix 1.

To ensure a successful change to multidisciplinary rounding, implementation barriers were explored and strategies developed to address these barriers were created. One obstacle in the high-acuity NICU was crowd control and noise abatement. This occurred most often when both teams were simultaneously rounding within the same hallway. During rounds, if the Doc team and the NNP team converged in the same hallway to round on different patients, the hallway could be filled with 20 or more people and mobile computer workstations, creating a traffic jam. This disrupted parent and ancillary staff movement as well as mobilization of any patient care equipment. This also limited the continuity and flow of rounds with nurses and respiratory therapists unable to participate in discussions with both teams simultaneously. A strategy was developed focusing on the flow and coordination of the 2 medical teams within the unit, with flexibility of both teams emphasized. It also resulted in lower noise levels and commotion in the hallways, thus decreasing disturbances for families and other ancillary staff.

Another concern was the slowing of rounds if the nurse or respiratory therapist was not present in the hallway due to other patient care responsibilities, such as off-unit diagnostic tests, procedures, or obstetric deliveries during rounding. To address this concern, daily morning individual hallway huddles prior to rounds were held. These 7:30 AM hallway huddles include the nurses and respiratory therapists caring for patients within the hallway. It allowed further coordination of team members, so if a nurse or therapist had to be absent from rounds, another member of the team was present to listen to rounds and update the plan on the rounding script. Hallway team members were alerted to the movement of a team to their hallway via a text message sent over the wireless handsets carried by unit staff. **Box 2** delineates coordination of team members.

Box 2
Coordination of team members

- As each team enters each hall, the rounding nurse or NNP team or fellow will call the front desk at x5-5255 to have the CCSR (Clinical Customer Service Representative) send out a page on the Ascom phones that "the Doc team will start rounding in Hallway 1 now" OR "the NNP team will start rounding in Hallway 2 now."
- That page will signal all nurses and RTs that have patients on that team in that hall to return in preparation for rounds. If assigned nurse are on break, it is expected that you return to your patients. Please plan breaks to not interfere with rounds.
- In the event that the assigned nurse or respiratory therapist is unable to be present for rounds. Use the huddle to make back-up plans to ensure rounds proceed smoothly (ie, if assigned nurse know the baby needs to go to MRI, make sure the teammates are aware that one of them will potentially have to listen for assigned nurse and update the last page of the rounding script, the PLAN).
- It is expected that assigned nurse and the other nurses in the hallway will work together to ensure that every nurse is able to present their babies during rounds (ie, if the nurse who needs to present is busy hanging blood, bottle feeding, etc., another nurse should do that task so that the nurse taking care of the patient can present rounds).

To ensure that rounds were conducted efficiently, it was decided that essential team members included the attending neonatologist, the assigned provider for the patient (either resident or NNP), bedside nurse, nutritionist, pharmacist, and parents if available. Rounds began on each patient with the resident or NNP giving a quick introduction of the patient, including name, gestational age, and primary medical problem. After this brief patient introduction, the nurse continued to present the remainder of the information, with respiratory therapists and nutritionists contributing. If the nurse was unable to be present, the resident or NNP presented that portion of information. After the presentation and development of the daily plan, the rounding script was updated by the day shift nurse to ensure the accuracy of information and contribute to the continuity of care, thus decreasing the change that parents received conflicting information. The rounding script then was used for the shift report and passed back to the assigned night shift nurse to be updated the next morning.

Moving forward, the education of the nursing staff was critical to the successful change in practice. A PowerPoint presentation was developed giving detailed instructions on each section of the rounding script. This presentation was extensive, consisting of more than 50 slides, detailing how to locate information in the electronic record and how to document and present the information on rounds. Extensive education was provided at staff meetings and in the monthly NICU newsletter, "The Preemie Press." The monthly NICU Journal Club featured the article written by Licata and colleagues,[6] detailing the successful implementation of interdisciplinary bedside rounds in a PICU setting. In addition to the PowerPoint presentation, flip charts in each hallway were provided as a quick resource guide. To provide visual demonstration, mock rounding presentations were videotaped and posted to YouTube (https://youtu.be/Mb5ydfMDuRI and https://youtu.be/InN2IsJP7Gg).

The accurate reporting of patient fluid status and intake and output resulted in a good deal of consternation for the night nursing staff that was responsible for the calculations. An extensive teaching tool was developed by one of the NNPs to assist the nursing staff in calculating the amounts accurately. For example, instruction was provided on how to determine and document total fluid intake and output, total caloric intake, glucose infusion rates, and ostomy output percentages. The importance of using the proper weight for the patient was also addressed. As in many NICUs, birthweight was used for the first week of life or until infants regained their birthweight. Critically ill infants often had a designated dry weight, which was used for medication dosing and fluid management if they had significant edema or other fluid balance issues. This was imperative for staff to understand, because the electronic medical record listed the last recorded weight for these calculations and could result in inaccurate medication dosing and intravenous fluid orders. Specific examples were given to help illustrate the concepts. **Box 3** and **Table 1** provide rounding tips.

The educational needs of the medical staff had to be considered during the rollout of multidisciplinary rounds. The concept of educational medical rounds, conducted at the patient bedside, has historically been associated with Johns Hopkins Hospital. This concept was first developed in the nineteenth century and has remained a respected tradition. Sir William Osler, the first physician-in-chief of the Johns Hopkins Hospital, established a system of medical education built on bringing medical students, interns, and residents to the actual bedside of the patient.[6] The term, *rounds*, is most likely based on the design of the original hospital building, currently known as the Billings Administration Building, which was built with octagonal wards, thus requiring the team to progress in a circular path around the ward to each patient bedside.[7] **Fig. 1** shows the physical room configuration.

Bedside rounds contribute to the medical education and hands-on learning of residents, fellows, and medical students. Medical staff expressed some concern that with the increased role of nurses and other team members during rounds the educational component of rounds for medical staff would be diminished. It was emphasized that participation of other team members would increase learning opportunities from staff with a different focus of expertise. Residents were still expected to present a detailed assessment and plan for each patient on their team, with deeper insight provided by nursing and other team members, so that a thoughtful and thorough plan of care could be developed.

As the time for rollout approached, nursing staff expressed a range of emotions. Many were excited and looked forward to the expanded role for nurses, whereas some nurses expressed apprehension and anxiety about speaking in front of a group, and others believed rounding was not within their job description. The nursing staff had a wide age range and varied experience levels, some nurses with less than 1 year's experience and others with more than 35 years of experience in the same NICU. There had been an attempt to implement a team approach to rounds several years prior, which had been met with opposition from nurses. The effort lacked a dedicated group of nursing staff to champion the cause and a medical leader willing to advocate for the role change. A few nurses spoke of boycotting the change; however, it was made clear by the NICU nurse manager that this evidence-based practice change was now part of the nursing role and participation was not optional. To ensure success, buy-in from all members of the team was crucial and the conversion required all nurses to participate.

Committee members worked extensively with individual nurses to increase their comfort level and decrease stage fright. As issues were raised, they were addressed proactively through the use of emails and frequently asked question sheets available throughout the unit. One week prior to the beginning of multidisciplinary rounding, rounding scripts were distributed and night shift nurses began filling out the rounding scripts and using them for shift report with a committee member available to provide assistance and answer any questions. On the day of rollout and continuing for the first few weeks thereafter, members of the development committee were made available to assist the day shift nursing staff before and during rounding. One team member

Box 3
Calculation tips

Calculating GIR

A quick way to figure up the GIR: multiply dextrose % × IV rate/hour × 0.167 ÷ weight in kilograms = GIR

Example: infant who weighs 1120 g is on D10 PN at 6 mL/h plus is on dopamine infusion at 0.3 mL/h, which is mixed in D5W.

PN (D10) = 10 × 6 × 0.167 ÷ 1.12 = GIR 8.9
Dopamine (D5) 5 × 0.3 × 0.167 ÷1.12 = GIR 0.22
8.9 + 0.22 = 9.12 total GIR

Say he also is has a UAC line with .45% sodium acetate + heparin at 1 mL/h (GIR 0 because no glucose) and lipids at 0.5 mL/h, and he is NPO. To calculate his projected total fluids per kilogram, add up the hourly rate of all his infusions, multiply by 24 h, and divide by his weight (6 + 1 + 0.3 + 0.5) × 24 ÷ 1.12 = 167 mL/kg.

Calculating total fluids—from all sources from midnight to midnight

Total fluid includes amounts from all sources from midnight to midnight: IV fluids, feedings, blood products, fluid boluses, etc.

Let's say a 1500-g baby was on PN at 3.5 mL/h and lipids at 0.5 mL/h and receiving feedings of breast milk 15 mL every 3 h. Total fluids would be 144 mL/kg/d.

3.5 + 0.5 = 4 mL/h 4 × 24 h = 96 mL/d from IV fluids

15 × 8 feedings a day = 120 mL/d

96 + 120 = 216 mL/d

216 ÷ 1.5 kg = 144 mL/kg/d

The weight used to calculate total fluids is the weight from prior to the 24-h total that is being assessed.

For example, Monday morning rounds total fluids are calculated from Sunday @0001 to Monday @0000. The weight used should be Saturday P shift's weight.

Make sure to check that all intake is charted. Sometimes feedings are accidently not charted and it seems that the baby's total fluids are low. Also make sure stools are marked under output information (stool occurrence). If they are only charted under stool assessment, they will not show up on the intake and output for the day.

Calculating ostomy output

Ostomy output is in milliliters. The Docs and GPS also like to know what the ostomy output is as a percentage of the intake. For example: if an infant has 42 mL of ostomy output and received feedings of 5 mL/h, the ostomy output is 35% of the enteral intake (PO/NG); 5 mL/h × 24 h = 120 mL of intake; 42 mL ÷ 120 = .35 or 35%. GPS will want to know how much output baby has had per kilogram. So if a baby weighs 2 kg, his ostomy output equals 21 mL/kg.

If you notice that an infant has lost more than 10% of his birthweight, make sure to mention it in rounds. The baby may need more fluid volume.

Calculating calories/kilogram/day—only used if baby is on full feeds

To calculate the number of calories a day a baby is receiving from his feedings, multiply the number of milliliters of formula the baby is receiving per day by the number of calories in 1 mL of formula and divide this number by the baby's weight in kilograms. Keep in mind that if someone enters the midnight bolus/bottle feed at 2340, it will add more volume to the totals, so it best to calculate it out yourself:

For example, if a baby weighs 1500 g and is receiving 28 mL of breast milk fortified to 24 cal/oz every 3 h, he would get a total of 224 mL of formula a day. His formula is 24 cal/oz, which is 0.8 cal/mL (24 cal/oz ÷ 30 mL in an ounce).

28 mL × 8 feedings/d = 224 mL

224 mL × 0.8 = 179.2 cal/d ÷ 1.5 kg = 119.4 kcal/kg/d

A quick reference of calories in each milliliter of formula or breast milk:

20 cal/oz = 0.67 cal/mL

22 cal/oz = 0.73 cal/mL

24 cal/oz = 0.8 cal/mL

26 cal/oz = 0.86 cal/mL

27 cal/oz = 0.9 cal/mL

30 cal/oz = 1 cal/mL

Note: We do this calculation of calories per day once baby has reached full-volume feeds.

Calculating urine output—mL/kg/d (MN to MN)

Total milliliters of urine output divided by 24 (hours) divided by yesterday's weight.

Abbreviations: D5/D5W, 5% Dextrose solution; D10, 10% Dextrose solution; GIR, glucose infusion rate; GPS, general pediatric surgery; IV, intravenous; NG, nasogastric; NPO, nothing by mouth; p, PM; PN, parenteral nutrition; UAC, umbilical arterial line.

was assigned to each rounding team to provide elbow-to-elbow support to the bedside nurses as they presented during rounds.

RESULTS

Approximately 18 months has elapsed since the changeover began, and nurses are now an integral part of multidisciplinary rounds. In the vast majority of instances, the bedside nurse is present and actively participates in rounds. Occasions do arise that require the nurse to be absent from the bedside during rounds, but strategies have been developed to assure the accurate communication of any changes or updates. Despite a good deal of angst, it has been successful but not without challenges. Over this same time frame, the unit has experienced an increase in both census and patient acuity, with the expansion of an innovative perinatal fetal therapy program. This has led to an increased workload for nurses in an already demanding environment. The rounding script has gone through multiple revisions, with adjustments reflecting the dynamic necessities of nurses, providers, patients, and families. Nurses are now sharing their unique and comprehensive knowledge of patients in addition to acting as advocates for patients and families. Some of the nurses who expressed the most hesitancy with the change have made the adjustment with ease, rounding on their patients as the expert caregivers they are. One veteran nurse who had been especially apprehensive prior to the rollout adopted to the change adeptly, becoming a resource for other nurses as well.

FUTURE IMPLICATIONS

It is obvious to participants that the unit as a whole has benefitted from the increased role of the nurse on rounds, but an effort should be made to quantify the benefit. Investigation to determine if the change in rounding structure has had an impact on patient safety and family satisfaction within the NICU is the next step in the process. A study to examine the rate of patient safety event reports pre-rollout and post-rollout would be informative as would a comparison of patient satisfaction survey results. Because previous studies have indicated that collaboration with medical teams and

Table 1
Calculation card

Glucose infusion rate	$\frac{(D\%)(IV\ rate)\ (0.167)}{Weight(kilograms)}$
Calories from feeds (kilocalories/kilogram/day) 20 = 0.67 22 = 0.73 24 = 0.8 27 = 0.9 30 = 1	$\frac{(Total\ volume\ of\ feeds\ in\ millilitres)\ (kcal\ of\ feed \div 30)}{Weight}$
Calories from dextrose solution (kilocalories/kilogram/day)	$\frac{(D\%)\ (IV\ rate)\ (0.816)}{Weight}$
Calories from PN/IL (kilocalories/kilogram/day)	$\frac{(Total\ calories\ on\ PN\ order\ report)}{Weight}$
Calories from PN/IL if rate changes (kilocalories/kilogram/day)	$\frac{(New\ PN\ or\ IL\ rate)\ (Total\ calories\ on\ order\ report)}{(Old\ PN\ or\ IL\ rate\ on\ order\ report)\ (Weight)}$
Ostomy output (milliliters/kilogram/day)	$\frac{(Total\ volume\ of\ stool\ in\ millilitres)}{Weight}$
Ostomy output % of PO/enteral intake Goal <35%	$\frac{(Total\ volume\ of\ stool\ in\ millilitres)}{(Total\ volume\ of\ feeds\ in\ millilitres)}$
Replogle/NG/OG output (milliliters/kilogram/day)	$\frac{(Total\ volume\ of\ output\ in\ millilitres)}{Weight}$
Heparin (unit/kilogram/day) Goal <70	$\frac{(Units/mL)\ (IV\ rate)\ (24)}{Weight}$

Abbreviations: D, Dextrose; GIR, glucose infusion rate; IL, intralipids or fats; IV, intravenous; NG, Naso-gastric; OG, oral-gastric; PN, parenteral nutrition; PO, By mouth; TEF, tracheoesophageal fistula; wt, weight.

Calculate all drips separately and add together.

Calories—calculate using what feeds/IV fluids they are on when you do your calculations (after 0600).

Replogle/NG/OG: calculate only if significant. Do not need to calculate if baby has TEF.

Use the most recent weight (kilograms) for everything, unless: baby <1 wk and losing weight (use birthweight) or baby is postoperative or extremely edematous (use dosing weight).

When in doubt, ask the residents/NNPs which weight they are using to calculate their fluids.

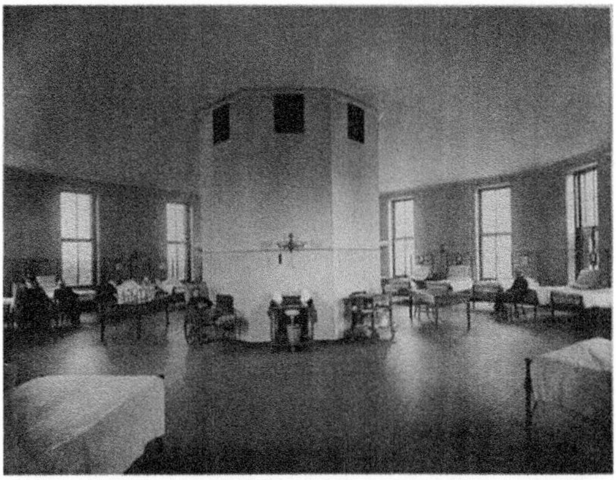

Fig. 1. Octagon ward: interior view. (*From* Medical Archives of The Johns Hopkins Medical Institutions. Collection, Item 184793. Available at: http://medicalarchives.jhmi.edu:8080.)

interdisciplinary relationships have been associated with higher levels of nursing job satisfaction,[5] it would also be insightful to study the impact on nursing job satisfaction.

ACKNOWLEDGMENTS

The authors would like to acknowledge all the members of the NICU Patient Satisfaction Committee: Eileen Conner, RN; Sue Culp, RN, NICU Nurse Manager; Susan Aucott, Medical Director of Johns Hopkins NICU; and all nursing and medical staff who went above and beyond to make this practice change possible.

REFERENCES

1. Shudy M, de Almeida ML, Ly S, et al. Impact of pediatric critical illness and injury on families: a systematic literature review. Pediatrics 2006;118(Suppl 3):S203–18.
2. Wills A, Wills J. I wish you knew. Pediatr Nurs 2009;35(5):318–21. Available at: CINAHL Plus with Full Text. Ipswich, MA. Accessed February 1, 2018.
3. Leonard M, Graham S, Bonacum D. The human factor: the critical importance of effective teamwork and communication in providing safe care. Qual Saf Health Care 2004;13:85–90.
4. Kalisch BJ, Lee H, Rochman M. Nursing staff teamwork and job satisfaction. J Nurs Manag 2010;18(8):938–47.
5. Gausvik C, Lautar A, Miller L, et al. Structured nursing communication on interdisciplinary acute care teams improves perceptions of safety, efficiency, understanding of care plan and teamwork as well as job satisfaction. J Multidiscip Healthc 2015;8:33–7.
6. Licata J, Aneja R, Kyper C, et al. A Foundation for patient safety: phase I implementation of interdisciplinary bedside rounds in the pediatric intensive care unit. Crit Care Nurse 2013;33:89091.
7. Osler W. The natural method of teaching the subject of medicine. JAMA 1901;36: 1673–6. History of Johns Hopkins Hospital, School of Medicine History. Obtained from The Johns Hopkins Medicine. Available at: https://www.hopkinsmedicine.org/Medicine/education/hstrainingprogram/overview/hx_jhh.html. Accessed January 8, 2018.

Standardized Feeding Protocols to Reduce Risk of Necrotizing Enterocolitis in Fragile Infants Born Premature or with Congenital Heart Disease

Implementation Science Needed

Sheila M. Gephart, PhD, RN[a,*], Emily F. Moore, RN, MSN, CPNP[b], Emory Fry, MD[c]

KEYWORDS

- Standardized feeding protocol • Neonate • Congenital heart disease
- Necrotizing enterocolitis • Clinical decision support • Implementation science

KEY POINTS

- Necrotizing enterocolitis is a devastating intestinal infection that develops after birth in fragile infants, especially those born very low birth weight or with congenital heart disease.
- Although NEC is serious and deadly, some risk factors for the disease are modifiable. Feeding using a structured approach to starting, stopping, advancing and fortifying feeding- especially when human milk is used- reduces NEC.
- Effectively implementing a feeding protocol to reduce NEC is supported by integrating it into electronic order sets, checking compliance through audit and feedback and making sure that all team members have access to the protocol.

Funding: Dr S.M. Gephart received funding from the Robert Wood Johnson Foundation Nurse Faculty Scholars Program (72112), the Agency for Healthcare Research and Quality (K08HS022908), and an express outreach award from the University of California, Los Angeles, Louise M. Darling Biomedical Library, headquarters for the National Network of Libraries of Medicine, Pacific Southwest Region (NNLM PSR). The content is solely the responsibility of the authors and does not necessarily represent the official views of the Agency for Healthcare Research and Quality, Robert Wood Johnson Foundation, or NNLM.
Disclosure: The authors have nothing to disclose.
[a] Community and Health Systems Science, College of Nursing, The University of Arizona, PO Box 210203, Tucson, AZ 85721, USA; [b] Regional cardiology program, Seattle Children's Hospital, 4800 Sand Point Way NE, Seattle, WA 98105, USA; [c] Cognitive Medical Systems, 9444 Waples Street, Suite 300, San Diego, CA 92121, USA
* Corresponding author.
E-mail address: gepharts@email.arizona.edu

Crit Care Nurs Clin N Am 30 (2018) 457–466
https://doi.org/10.1016/j.cnc.2018.07.003
ccnursing.theclinics.com

One of the chief threats to the health of fragile infants surviving early life is NEC. NEC is a devastating intestinal infection afflicting primarily very-low-birth-weight (VLBW, ie, <1500 g) infants, affecting 9000 infants and resulting in the death of about 3000 annually in the United States.[1] NEC is thought to arise from multiple factors that assault the infant, who is unable to mount a healthy immune response. NEC occurs in the context of excessive mucosal inflammation, underdeveloped intestinal mucosa, disrupted bacterial colonization, ischemic-hypoxic injury in some, and enteral feeding in most.[2] NEC has several risk factors.[2–4] Although rare among term infants, infants with CHD, intrauterine growth restriction, or cocaine exposure are at risk.[5,6] Formula feeding is one of the chief modifiable NEC risk factors.[7,8]

Promoting human milk (HM), especially mother's own milk, reduces NEC in preterm groups.[7] HM has benefits for the fragile infant exceeding the need for nutrition and tackling the primary challenge in the ill newborn: inflammation out of control. Many describe HM for preterm infants as medicine, even calling it, "*Liquid Gold.*"[9] One health economist estimated if the United States increases HM exposure to optimal levels, $27 million in direct care and $1.5 billion could be saved and could translate to 928 fewer NEC cases and 121 lives saved.[10]

Most NEC research has focused on the preterm population; however, when children with CHD develop NEC, they have very high mortality. For CHD NEC survivors, their nutritional capacity diminishes and leads to long-term health impacts.[11] It is possible that NEC prevention approaches effective in preterm populations will be useful for the CHD population. Although the last 3 decades generated intense focus on cause and antecedents of NEC, only modest improvements in NEC burden have been made.[12] The purpose of this article is to bridge the gap between recommended and actual care using standardized feeding protocols (SFPs) (**Table 1**).

Table 1
Definitions

Necrotizing enterocolitis (NEC)	Death of intestine that is the end result of an exaggerated and dysregulated inflammatory process, abnormal colonization of bacteria, a fragile and incompetent mucosal barrier, and intolerance to enteral feeding (especially bovine products)
Spontaneous intestinal perforation (SIP)	Spontaneous rupture of a localized area of the intestine, often the terminal ileum, especially in infants <27-wk' gestation in first 1–2 wk of life. Differentiating SIP from NEC reveals an isolated perforation that does not involve widespread intestinal ischemia and mucosal destruction
Congenital heart disease (CHD)	Heart problem present at birth caused by abnormal fetal development. Can involve walls, valves, or heart structure. Classified as acyanotic or cyanotic
Acyanotic heart disease	Heart disease involving left-to-right shunting and increased pulmonary blood flow
Cyanotic heart disease	Heart disease that leads to central cyanosis due to insufficient pulmonary blood flow or mixing of the red and blue blood in systemic circulation
Standardized feeding protocol (SFP)	Written criteria to initiate, advance, stop (with definitions and approaches to handle feeding intolerance), and fortify feeding
Feeding intolerance	Disrupted digestion, common in preterm infants who have slow peristalsis, small stomachs, and may be critically ill. May include emesis, gastric residuals >25%–50% of previous feeding volume, abdominal distension, and/or increased abdominal girth

NECROTIZING ENTEROCOLITIS PATHOPHYSIOLOGY IN PREMATURE INFANT

Hackam and Caplan[13] proposed that NEC develops because of several factors that interact and predispose a neonate who may also have genetic vulnerability. An underdeveloped and hyperinflammatory intestinal epithelium common to premature infants overexpresses toll-like receptor 4 (TL4) more than in developed (ie, term) epithelium when NEC occurs. They argue bacteria colonization in the gut activates TLR4 expression if pathogenic bacteria are most prevalent (especially gram-negative *proteobacteria*) compared with beneficial bacteria. TLR expression with dysbiosis leads to a compromised gut barrier, where activated TL4 leads to mucosal injury, poor mucosal repair, and bacteria translocation across the intestinal lumen followed by vasoconstriction and death in the intestine characteristic of NEC. Essential to turning down TL4 activation is breast milk enteral feeding, which inhibits TL4 signaling with its many growth factors (especially epidermal) and highly bioactive oligosaccharides. Breast milk also provides bacteria competing with pathogenic bacteria to prevent overgrowth. In some neonates, genetic alterations to TLR4-signalling or pathways involved in restraining TLR4 produce NEC susceptibility.[13]

To diagnose NEC, there must be both clinical and radiologic signs according to common definitions from the *International Classification of Diseases, Tenth Revision* and the Vermont-Oxford Network (VON). NEC clinical presentation includes systemic signs like increasing apnea or bradycardia, oxygen desaturation, general lethargy or irritability, discolored abdomen (red or dusky are most worrisome), increasing abdominal girth or gastric residual volumes, vomiting, bloody stool, and abdominal distension.[14,15] Late clinical signs include decreasing platelet counts, increased ventilator requirements, a taut, red, or dusky abdomen, and bloody stool. Aradiograph or ultrasound provides confirmatory evidence for NEC when pneumatosis is present. When NEC is severe, radiographs and ultrasound will also show pneumoperitoneum or portal air.[16] Some researchers argue these are not specific enough to distinguish NEC from other newborn acquired intestinal diseases and propose alternative definitions.[17,18]

In determining whether an infant has "NEC," it is critical to differentiate "NEC" from other conditions affecting the neonatal intestine. One primary condition causing perforation of the gut but without widespread necrosis and infection is spontaneous intestinal perforation (SIP).[19] SIP presents typically with pneumoperitoneum but not pneumatosis. Some argue SIP has similar gastrointestinal presentation to NEC without the symptoms of systemic infection and metabolic derangement.

The "2-out-of-3 rule" was recently proposed to guide bedside diagnosis of preterm NEC.[15] In this definition, preterm is less than 36 weeks' gestational age at birth and the typical day of life that NEC emerges compared with SIP, as shown in a nomogram published by the Pediatrix medical group.[19] If an infant has abdominal distension, bloody stools, and/or ileus and has 2 of the 3 following conditions: (1) pneumatosis and/or portal air detected via abdominal radiograph or ultrasound, (2) persistent consumption of platelets (<150,000 platelets within 3 days after diagnosis), and (3) the postmenstrual age at onset is consistent with NEC vs SIP, they can be diagnosed as "NEC." Patients are excluded from this definition of preterm NEC if they (1) have SIP confirmed at surgery, (2) have congenital anomalies, are being fed less than 80 mL/kg/d, or (3) are greater than 36 weeks' gestation.[15]

NECROTIZING ENTEROCOLITIS PATHOPHYSIOLOGY IN ISCHEMIC INJURY WITH HYPOPERFUSION IN CONGENITAL HEART DISEASE

CHD is commonly broken into 2 categories: cyanotic and acyanotic. Babies with acyanotic heart disease often have a left-to-right shunting defect, such as an atrial or ventricular septal defect. These defects have too much pulmonary blood flow. Babies are at risk for developing congestive heart failure and often treated with diuretics.

Hypoplastic Left Heart Syndrome (HLHS) is a common single-ventricle diagnosis placing the infant at high risk for NEC.[20] Treatment is complex and multifactorial and requires lifelong dedication by patients and their families. To understand HLHS complexity, it is essential to understand the basic pathophysiology of this anomaly, which is rare and life threatening and characterized by underdevelopment of the left ventricle and systemic outflow tract obstruction. The Centers for Disease Control and Prevention estimates that 960 babies are born with HLHS each year in the United States.[21] In HLHS, the patient has an underdeveloped left ventricle, aorta, mitral valve, and aortic valve requiring multiple surgical palliations.[20,22] Beginning in the first few days of life, the patient undergoes first surgical intervention, known as stage 1 palliation. The goal of stage 1 is to provide systemic-to-pulmonary shunt, ultimately improving systemic blood flow and oxygenation. The surgical process for creating this shunt is done by connecting the pulmonary artery to the neonate's aorta and creating pulmonary blood flow by a systemic-to-pulmonary shunt or by a shunt from the right ventricle to the pulmonary artery.[23]

Patients with single-ventricle cyanotic heart disease have both pulmonary and systemic blood flow supplied from one pumping chamber. This ventricle has a significant volume load, which can increase energy expenditure. These infants typically need surgery within the first days of life. Because of decreased blood flow to the gut, these infants are at an increased risk for developing NEC along with several other complications, including prolonged hospitalizations, delayed healing, poor nutrition, feeding difficulties, and vocal cord injury.[24]

STANDARDIZED FEEDING PROTOCOLS

Most clinicians would say breast milk is important for all infants and would identify it as an NEC prevention strategy.[25] However, before 2005, few neonatal clinicians would identify a standardized approach to feeding via a unit-adopted SFP to be protective against NEC. An SFP is a structured protocol that ordering clinicians agree to follow specifying criteria to initiate, advance, stop, and fortify feeding. It should include a protocol for identifying and managing feeding intolerance. In 2005, a meta-analysis showed SFPs reduce NEC risk by 29% in VLBW infants and about 87% for infants less than 2500 g[26] Around the same time, the VON led an initiative to spread better practices for neonatal care. One of the VON groups addressed feeding practices, recommending adoption of a unit-based consistent approach through an SFP.[27,28] In 2015, an interdisciplinary group of experts reviewed NEC prevention evidence to answer key questions on *how* changes could be implemented feasibly in practice through an initiative called "NEC-Zero."[29] The NEC-Zero SFP subgroup reevaluated SFP evidence since the 2005 meta-analysis to include 9 new studies in infants less than 1500 g. Care of infants outside of that population, or if studies included explicitly multi-faceted quality improvement work, was excluded. Among 4755 infants (<1500 g) included from 9 studies, SFPs conferred a 67% reduced odds for NEC (odds ratio 0.33, 95% confidence interval 0.17, 0.65).[29] Shortly before their results were published, Jasani and Patole[30] published their meta-analysis addressing the effect of SFPs on *all* infants at risk for NEC. Most of the 15 studies included infants less than 2500 g or less than 1500 g (N = 18,160 infants) but did not include studies with CHD-affected neonates or conduct a subgroup analysis for the infants less than 1500 g. However, they also showed 78% reduced NEC risk when a unit adopted an SFP (P<.00001).[30]

Key Features of Effective Standardized Feeding Protocols

Details of effective feeding regimens have been shown to vary widely, although effective SFPs include duration of minimal enteral feeding, for example, trophic feeds, prioritize breast milk, avoid fortification until meeting minimum volume, and outline criteria for holding feeding or for determining intolerance to feeding. To promote the maturation of the gut, early feeding initiation is important. Prioritizing fresh mother's milk is important to supply the bioactive benefits of breast milk after the colostrum is given.

Period of trophic feeding

Most of the effective SFPs include a period of small-volume feedings (10–20 mL/kg/d) lasting between 2 and 5 days and starting by 72 hours of age.[30,31] This practice followed results of a study by Berseth and colleagues[32] showing fast advancement without trophic feeds led to more NEC compared with including a period of trophic feeding.

Feeding advancement

An SFP should include a schedule for the rate at which feeding will be advanced and how often (eg, once or twice a day). SFPs that are effective in high-risk populations are published.[33,34] Schedules to guide the feeding advancement have also been found to be very helpful. A resource for feeding schedules is available from the Supporting Premature Infant Nutrition program (https://health.ucsd.edu/specialties/obgyn/maternity/newborn/nicu/spin/staff/Pages/tables.aspx).[35]

Cause for feeding interruptions

When framing SFP, clinicians need to identify when to interrupt feeding, how to define feeding intolerance, what algorithms to detect it, and how to restart feeding when interrupted. Some may elect to interrupt feeding during periods when mesenteric perfusion is reduced (eg, on inotropic medication for hypotension, if a transfusion is given, when septic, for patent ductus arteriosus that is severe or during indomethacin therapy). Evidence is inconsistent on how best to handle such situations.

Management of fortification

Fortification of HM is standard of care in the United States, although less common elsewhere.[36] Fortification begins when a minimum volume (typically >80 mL/kg/d) is met. Until recently, only bovine-based fortifiers were available. Donor HM-derived fortifiers are now available.

STANDARDIZED FEEDING PROTOCOLS IN INFANTS WITH HEART DISEASE

CHD is a universal concern and risk factor for NEC. Several studies identify prematurity and low birth weight magnifying NEC risk in newborns with CHD.[37] Feeding dysfunction occurs commonly, especially in those with ductal-dependent heart disease. These feeding dysfunctions have the potential to impact postoperative recovery, growth, and long-term outcomes, including long term feeding difficulties.[24]

There is no precise and prescribed "best" feeding practice to modify risk for NEC in infants with CHD. However, multiple groups recommend using SFPs. Consequently, recommendations for feeding are synthesized from literature. Some studies suggest an enteral feeding algorithm may be effective in decreasing the NEC prevalence in postoperative infants with CHD. A survey by the National Pediatric Cardiology Quality Improvement Collaborative (NPC-QIC) found SFPs are specific not only to institution but to practitioner.[38] In the absence of global consensus about a "best" approach, some debate the benefits of standardized feedings both preoperatively and postoperatively.

There are multiple benefits to early preoperative feeding such as enhanced gastrointestinal maturation, reduced time that parenteral nutrition is needed, better caloric density fed overall and better achievement of postoperative feeding goals. Similarly, studies have shown early enteral nutrition implementation leads to improved nutritional outcomes, shortened duration on mechanical ventilation, lowered infection rates, improved wound healing, decreased length of stay, and reduced mortality in critically ill patients.[11,39,40]

Delayed enteral feeding should be limited to low cardiac output states such as in neonates with ductal-dependent cardiac lesions or during treatment with extracorporeal membrane oxygenation. Feeding should be initiated with caution in the presence of an umbilical artery catheter. Feeding may be held due to sudden change in vital signs or increase in respiratory support, initiated inotropic support, noted gastrointestinal distress, or poor systemic output. In one study by Boston Children's Hospital, SFP implementation was done with clear definition of when to stop feeding.[41] They found that they decreased feeding interruptions (3 after the SFP vs 51 before, $P<.0001$) and were successful shortening the median time to reach energy goals from 4 days to 1 day ($P<.001$), and more infants met their energy goals (99% post-SFP vs 31% pre-SFP, $P = .01$).[41]

Postoperative patients with CHD are at risk for feeding problems, such as poor feeding skills, aspiration, vocal cord injury, gastroesophageal reflux, delayed gastric emptying, growth delays, feeding intolerance, and NEC. Patients who experienced decreased or low blood flow to their gut both preoperatively and intraoperatively are especially at risk because feeds are initiated in the postoperative period. If feeds are introduced, even at trophic rates/volumes, the gut is more likely to tolerate enteral feeds postoperatively.[42]

Implementation Science of Effective Standardized Feeding Protocols

When adopting an SFP, the authors recommend units integrate them into electronic or printed order sets, use feeding schedules, communicate to all clinical members, and conduct compliance audits with feedback to clinicians. Adopting SFP requires a multidisciplinary team, and most effective SFPs involved physicians, neonatal nurse practitioners, nurses, and dietitians at a minimum. Including parents in the team is best practice because they know their own baby best and are poised to watch for developing feeding complications. In infants with CHD who may go home between surgeries, it is critical to teach parents about feeding intolerance and NEC warning signs.

Implementation science is the study of how, why, and when effective practices are adopted in clinical settings and what strategies are most effective for consistent use. In the neonatal intensive care unit (NICU), work is chaotic, critical, and complex. Simple tools like SFPs may be triaged as less important while addressing other more immediately urgent concerns. Electronic medical record systems can be useful for implementing SFPs, although to the authors' knowledge, are underutilized. The Cerner electronic health record (EHR) has a fairly well developed Feeding Advance tool, but its implementation in practice has been sparse. The authors are unaware of SFPs integration on other EMR vendors. The authors' team created logic diagrams and rule-base to integrate SFPs into EMRs agnostic to any particular system. More information is available upon request.

Clinical decision support (CDS) reminders are effective across settings to improve adherence to recommended care, particularly for screening and prevention.[43] CDS to remind clinicians of gastric residual volumes are over a threshold or an infant is due for advance in volume are underutilized based on a survey the authors did in 2015 of US NICUs (Sheila M. Gephart, et al, personal communication, 2018). CDS to guide nursing decision-making at the bedside is underdeveloped and understudied overall.[44] CDS could be used to automate feeding intolerance algorithms or to clear the feeding schedule for an infant. The authors' team has tools available for CDS that could be useful to units wishing to streamline SFP development or automation.

While initiating an institutional-specific protocol for feeding in infants with CHD, the second author identified implementation concerns. Reports from the National Pediatric Cardiology Quality Improvement Collaborative were referenced and used to inform the protocol.[24] Given that infants with CHD are some of the most fragile and critically ill patients, an attempt to achieve balance between optimizing growth and maintaining safety was made. A standardized approach toward feeding was coupled with careful monitoring of hemodynamic status and feeding tolerance. Bedside nurses received thorough education and training regarding feeding assessment and tolerance. As a teaching hospital, all fellows were also educated regarding the protocol. After education, the protocol went "live." The unit-specific dietician tracked all patients placed on the protocol. With close monitoring, Seattle Children's was able to significantly decrease NEC in infants with CHD or "catch" NEC cases still in the early stages. When NEC was identified, a prompt surgical referral was made and infants at risk were treated for medical NEC with bowel rest and antibiotics. (Emily Moore, personal communication, 2018).

Next Steps in Practice and Research

In 2010, leading NEC researchers proposed if all NICUs were to adopt HM feeding and an SFP, NEC incidence could be cut in half.[45] To do so would take collective clinical will to break the inertia and dismantle beliefs around the inevitability of NEC. These words were not just hopeful words for all 3 authors had witnessed dramatic reductions in NEC in the units they covered: from Louisiana to Utah and Ohio. In 2013, the lead author reviewed evidence for SFPs in a paper titled, "Preventing Necrotizing enterocolitis with feeding protocols: not only impossible but imperative."[31] Although the title was somewhat ill accepted at the time, clinicians have shifted their practice using the protocols and the algorithm proposed in that paper. What is missing is the gap between what is *recommended* and what is *done* in practice. When SFPs are adopted, they may not be communicated widely to all staff, may leave out the critical piece of a feeding intolerance algorithm, or may simply be inconsistently followed. To close that gap, strategies such as using implementation science methods are needed. Using electronic strategies from the EHR, reminders to clinicians via CDS and leveraging algorithms to define and interpret feeding intolerance can all be useful.

Although shown to be effective, it is not clear which SFP is best, and comparative effectiveness studies are needed. In infants with CHD, more research is needed to show the effect of SFPs on nutritional outcomes and NEC. It is also unclear how best to engage parents in the process. In conclusion, SFPs are simple and low risk, and in more than 18,000 infants reduced NEC.

ACKNOWLEDGMENTS

The authors thank the NEC-Zero working group for their work in 2015 to review evidence about feeding protocols and propose implementation strategies.

REFERENCES

1. National Institute of Child Health and Human Development. How many infants are affected or at risk of necrotizing enterocolitis (NEC)? 2017. Available at: www.nichd.nih.gov. Accessed December 20, 2017.

2. Gephart SM, McGrath JM, Effken JA, et al. Necrotizing enterocolitis risk: state of the science. Adv Neonatal Care 2012;12(2):77–87 [quiz: 88–9].
3. Samuels N, van de Graaf RA, de Jonge RCJ, et al. Risk factors for necrotizing enterocolitis in neonates: a systematic review of prognostic studies. BMC Pediatr 2017;17(1):105.
4. Gephart SM. Validating a neonatal risk index to predict necrotizing enterocolitis. Tucson (AZ): University of Arizona; 2012.
5. Ostlie DJ, Spilde TL, St Peter SD, et al. Necrotizing enterocolitis in full-term infants. J Pediatr Surg 2003;38(7):1039–42.
6. Lambert DK, Christensen RD, Henry E, et al. Necrotizing enterocolitis in term neonates: data from a multihospital health-care system. J Perinatol 2007;27(7): 437–43.
7. Sullivan S, Schanler RJ, Kim JH, et al. An exclusively human milk-based diet is associated with a lower rate of necrotizing enterocolitis than a diet of human milk and bovine milk-based products. J Pediatr 2010;156(4):562–7.e1.
8. Quigley M, McGuire W. Formula versus donor breast milk for feeding preterm or low birth weight infants. Cochrane Database Syst Rev 2014;(4):CD002971.
9. Pletsch D, Ulrich C, Angelini M, et al. Mothers' "liquid gold": a quality improvement initiative to support early colostrum delivery via oral immune therapy (OIT) to premature and critically ill newborns. Nurs Leadersh (Tor Ont) 2013;26(Spec No 2013):34–42.
10. Colaizy TT, Bartick MC, Jegier BJ, et al. Impact of optimized breastfeeding on the costs of necrotizing enterocolitis in extremely low birthweight infants. J Pediatr 2016;175:100–5.e2.
11. Karpen HE. Nutrition in the cardiac newborns: evidence-based nutrition guidelines for cardiac newborns. Clin Perinatol 2016;43(1):131–45.
12. Horbar JD, Edwards EM, Greenberg LT, et al. Variation in performance of neonatal intensive care units in the United States. JAMA Pediatr 2017;171(3): e164396.
13. Hackam D, Caplan M. Necrotizing enterocolitis: pathophysiology from a historical context. Semin Pediatr Surg 2018;27(1):11–8.
14. Gephart SM, Fleiner M, Kijewski A. The ConNECtion between abdominal signs and necrotizing enterocolitis in infants 501 to 1500 g. Adv Neonatal Care 2017; 17(1):53–64.
15. Gephart SM, Gordon PV, Penn AH, et al. Changing the paradigm of defining, detecting, and diagnosing NEC: perspectives on Bell's stages and biomarkers for NEC. Semin Pediatr Surg 2018;27(1):3–10.
16. Di Napoli A, Di Lallo D, Perucci CA, et al. Inter-observer reliability of radiological signs of necrotising enterocolitis in a population of high-risk newborns. Paediatr Perinat Epidemiol 2004;18(1):80–7.
17. Gordon P, Christensen R, Weitkamp JH, et al. Mapping the new world of necrotizing enterocolitis (NEC): review and opinion. EJ Neonatol Res 2012;2(4):145–72.
18. Gordon PV, Swanson JR. Necrotizing enterocolitis is one disease with many origins and potential means of prevention. Pathophysiology 2014;21(1):13–9.
19. Gordon PV, Clark R, Swanson JR, et al. Can a national dataset generate a nomogram for necrotizing enterocolitis onset? J Perinatol 2014;34(10):732–5.
20. Harrison AM, Davis S, Reid JR, et al. Neonates with hypoplastic left heart syndrome have ultrasound evidence of abnormal superior mesenteric artery perfusion before and after modified Norwood procedure. Pediatr Crit Care Med 2005;6(4):445–7.

21. CDC. Congenital Heart Defects 2016. Available at: https://www.cdc.gov/ncbddd/heartdefects/hlhs.html. Accessed December 20, 2017.
22. Miller TA, Minich LL, Lambert LM, et al. Abnormal abdominal aorta hemodynamics are associated with necrotizing enterocolitis in infants with hypoplastic left heart syndrome. Pediatr Cardiol 2014;35(4):616–21.
23. Everett AD, Scott D, Lim MD. Illustrated field guide to congenital heart disease and repair. Charlottesville (VA): Scientific Software Solutions; 2007.
24. Slicker J, Hehir DA, Horsley M, et al. Nutrition algorithms for infants with hypoplastic left heart syndrome; birth through the first interstage period. Congenit Heart Dis 2013;8(2):89–102.
25. Gephart SM, Poole SN, Crain DR. Qualitative description of neonatal expert perspectives about necrotizing enterocolitis risk. Newborn Infant Nurs Rev 2014;14(3):124–30.
26. Patole SK, de Klerk N. Impact of standardised feeding regimens on incidence of neonatal necrotising enterocolitis: a systematic review and meta-analysis of observational studies. Arch Dis Child Fetal Neonatal Ed 2005;90(2):F147–51.
27. Kuzma-O'Reilly B, Duenas ML, Greecher C, et al. Evaluation, development and implementation of potentially better practices in neonatal intensive care nutrition. Pediatrics 2003;111(4):e461–70.
28. Hanson C, Sundermeier J, Dugick L, et al. Implementation, process, and outcomes of nutrition best practices for infants <1500 g. Nutr Clin Pract 2011;26(5):614–24.
29. Gephart SM, Hanson C, Wetzel CM, et al. NEC-zero recommendations from scoping review of evidence to prevent and foster timely recognition of necrotizing enterocolitis. Matern Health Neonatol Perinatol 2017;3:23.
30. Jasani B, Patole S. Standardized feeding regimen for reducing necrotizing enterocolitis in preterm infants: an updated systematic review. J Perinatol 2017;37(7):827–33.
31. Gephart SM, Hanson CK. Preventing necrotizing enterocolitis with standardized feeding protocols: not only possible, but imperative. Adv Neonatal Care 2013;13(1):48–54.
32. Berseth CL, Bisquera JA, Paje VU. Prolonging small feeding volumes early in life decreases the incidence of necrotizing enterocolitis in very low birth weight infants. Pediatrics 2003;111(3):529–34.
33. McCallie KR, Lee HC, Mayer O, et al. Improved outcomes with a standardized feeding protocol for very low birth weight infants. J Perinatol 2011;31(Suppl 1):S61–7.
34. Patel AL, Trivedi S, Bhandari NP, et al. Reducing necrotizing enterocolitis in very low birth weight infants using quality-improvement methods. J Perinatol 2014;34(11):850–7.
35. Kim JH. Necrotizing enterocolitis: the road to zero. Semin Fetal Neonatal Med 2014;19(1):39–44.
36. Battersby C, Longford N, Mandalia S, et al. Incidence and enteral feed antecedents of severe neonatal necrotising enterocolitis across neonatal networks in England, 2012-13: a whole-population surveillance study. Lancet Gastroenterol Hepatol 2017;2(1):43–51.
37. Radman M, Mack R, Barnoya J, et al. The effect of preoperative nutritional status on postoperative outcomes in children undergoing surgery for congenital heart defects in San Francisco (UCSF) and Guatemala City (UNICAR). J Thorac Cardiovasc Surg 2014;147(1):442–50.

38. Slicker J, Sables-Baus S, Lambert LM, et al. Perioperative feeding approaches in single ventricle infants: a survey of 46 centers. Congenit Heart Dis 2016;11(6): 707–15.
39. del Castillo SL, McCulley ME, Khemani RG, et al. Reducing the incidence of necrotizing enterocolitis in neonates with hypoplastic left heart syndrome with the introduction of an enteral feed protocol. Pediatr Crit Care Med 2010;11(3): 373–7.
40. Braudis NJ, Curley MAQ, Beaupre K, et al. Enteral feeding algorithm for infants with hypoplastic left heart syndrome poststage I palliation. Pediatr Crit Care Med 2009;10(4):460–6.
41. Hamilton S, McAleer DM, Ariagno K, et al. A stepwise enteral nutrition algorithm for critically ill children helps achieve nutrient delivery goals*. Pediatr Crit Care Med 2014;15(7):583–9.
42. Toms R, Jackson KW, Dabal RJ, et al. Preoperative trophic feeds in neonates with hypoplastic left heart syndrome. Congenit Heart Dis 2015;10(1):36–42.
43. Bright TJ, Wong A, Dhurjati R, et al. Effect of clinical decision-support systems: a systematic review. Ann Intern Med 2012;157(1):29–43.
44. Dunn Lopez K, Gephart SM, Raszewski R, et al. Integrative review of clinical decision support for registered nurses in acute care settings. J Am Med Inform Assoc 2017;24(2):441–50.
45. Christensen RD, Gordon PV, Besner GE. Can we cut the incidence of necrotizing enterocolitis in half–today? Fetal Pediatr Pathol 2010;29(4):185–98.

Neonatal Hypoglycemia

Is There a Sweet Spot?

Mary L. Puchalski, DNP, APRN, CNS, NNP-BC[a,b,*],
Terri L. Russell, DNP, APRN, NNP-BC[a,b],
Kristine A. Karlsen, PhD, APRN, NNP-BC[c,d]

KEYWORDS

- Hypoglycemia • Neonatal hypoglycemia • Glucose • Hyperinsulinemia • Neonate • LGA • IDM • SGA

KEY POINTS

- Glucose is vital for normal cellular metabolism and is the major energy substrate for brain metabolism; therefore, a continuous supply of glucose is essential for well-being.
- The human brain is highly vulnerable to injury when deprived of an adequate supply of glucose. Hypoglycemia during childhood is especially impactful because the brain is dynamically developing.
- Glucose availability is determined not solely by glucose concentrations (or measured level) but also by perfusion and glucose utilization.
- Knowing newborns with recurrent hypoglycemia may not be identified with intermittent monitoring underscores the importance of establishing a considerable margin of safety when establishing treatment thresholds.
- Signs and symptoms of neonatal hypoglycemia often mimic sepsis, brain injury, drug withdrawal, metabolic derangements, and/or respiratory distress.
- Transient perinatal stress hyperinsulinemia has been identified as a condition that may exacerbate hypoglycemia in any newborn already at risk for hypoglycemia.

INTRODUCTION

> *Biochemists draw the map of the roads, clinical investigators try to measure the traffic along them and the practicing clinician decides on which road to go…*
> *—J.C. Waterlow and A.J.W. Sim, as cited by Mehta[1(pF65)]*

Disclosure: The authors have nothing to disclose.
[a] Ann & Robert H. Lurie Children's Hospital of Chicago, Division of Neonatology, 25 East Chicago Avenue, Chicago, IL 60611, USA; [b] Department of Women, Children, and Family Health Science, University of Illinois at Chicago, 845 South Damen Avenue, M/C 802, Chicago, IL 60612, USA; [c] The S.T.A.B.L.E. Program, 3070 Rasmussen Road, Suite 120, Park City, UT 84098, USA; [d] Primary Children's Hospital, Neonatal Intensive Care Unit, 100 Mario Capecchi Drive, Salt Lake City, UT 84113, USA
* Corresponding author. Ann & Robert H. Lurie Children's Hospital of Chicago, Division of Neonatology, 225 East Chicago Avenue, Chicago, IL 60611.
E-mail address: marynnp@gmail.com

Crit Care Nurs Clin N Am 30 (2018) 467–480
https://doi.org/10.1016/j.cnc.2018.07.004 ccnursing.theclinics.com

Neonatal hypoglycemia (NH) is the most common metabolic issue in the newborn,[2–5] occurring in as many as 19% of infants overall,[6] and up to 51% of infant considered at-risk for NH.[7] The newborn with NH is unable to make the metabolic adaptation after birth to either maintain an adequate circulating concentration of glucose, use an alternate fuel to supply the body's organs, and/or to adapt to enteral nutrition. It is essential to maintain blood glucose (BG) levels because it is the only nutrient that can be supplied in sufficient quantities to the retina, germinal epithelium of the gonads, and most importantly, the brain, for utilization as an energy source. Current evidence provides a strong correlation between neuroglycopenia (impaired brain function due to low BG levels in the brain), and subsequent adverse neurologic sequelae.[2,8–17] Thus, assessment for and treatment of NH are critically important measures to prevent brain injury.[18]

Although screening at-risk newborns for NH to avoid adverse outcomes is now standard practice,[19–22] there is no consensus regarding what level of BG constitutes "clinically significant" hypoglycemia: a controversy that has raged for decades.[2,5,20,21,23] Furthering the dilemma is the fact that not all infants with a low BG are symptomatic due to immaturity of the neonatal brain and other factors that are not well understood.[4,24–26] In addition, screening involves the not insignificant pain of a needle stick and may interfere with opportunities for maternal bonding.[27] For the bedside clinician who strives to "above all, do no harm," all of this results in a quandary regarding which infants to treat.

DEFINITION OF HYPOGLYCEMIA

The term "hypoglycemia" was coined in the late nineteenth century, derived from the Greek words "hypo," meaning below or under, "glykys," meaning sweet, and "haima" (blood), -meaning a decreased level of sugar in the blood.[28] Although the first recognized occurrence of low neonatal BG was made in 1911,[29,30] asymptomatic hypoglycemia was not a cause of concern through the 1970s. Newborns routinely were not fed for 6 to 12 hours after birth due to the effect of routine general anesthesia for deliveries.[30–32] In addition, it was thought that premature infants could tolerate lower BG levels than term infants.[33] Maintaining a BG >40 mg/dL (2.2 mmol/L) did not become the accepted standard until the late 1980s.[9,34]

In 2011, the American Academy of Pediatrics (AAP) published a clinical report, "*Postnatal Homeostasis in Late Preterm and Term Infants*," intended to provide screening and management guidelines for NH in "at-risk" newborns who did not require neonatal intensive care: late preterm (LPT, between 24 and 36-6/7 weeks' gestation), small or large for gestational age (SGA, LGA), and infants of diabetic mothers (IDM).[19] This report includes proposed BG treatment thresholds well below those used by other industrialized nations[34,35] and were not based on evidence of neurologic safety, but rather a "pragmatic approach to a controversial issue where evidence was lacking but guidance was needed."[19(p575)] Nevertheless, many clinicians have since adopted the treatment thresholds and recommendations presented in this clinical report, as they are perceived as an "AAP Guideline."

The Pediatric Endocrine Society (PES) published recommendations for the evaluation and management of persistent hypoglycemia.[21] In contrast to the AAP's focus on transitional hypoglycemia, the PES recommends maintaining the plasma glucose concentration close to the mean for a healthy newborn in the first 24 hours of life and above the level where neuroglycopenic symptoms appear in older children and adults, greater than 50 mg/dL (2.8 mmol/L). After 48 hours of age, the plasma glucose should be maintained greater than 60 mg/dL (3.3 mmol/L). The PES identifies newborns "at-risk" for NH as: LGA (with or without maternal diabetes), preterm or postmature infants, IDM, perinatally stressed, and symptomatic of NH. They also warn about infants with suspected congenital hypoglycemic disorders and emphasize the importance of assuring NH is completely resolved before their discharge.

Other BG values without strong scientific data have been provided in the medical literature, and yet the exact definition of NH remains elusive, complicated, and controversial. The question and debate continue: "How low is too low and for how long?"[36(p10)] To date, a single BG value that predicts outcomes has not been identified. This is especially true for infants considered "at risk" for NH but healthy enough to feed.[9,10,23,37–40] Complicating this clinical enigma is the lack of an identified plasma glucose value that correlates with both symptoms of hypoglycemia and adverse neurologic sequelae.[2,41] Furthermore, a recent study found that infants with recurrent hypoglycemia may not be identified with intermittent monitoring, underscoring the importance of establishing a considerable margin of safety when establishing treatment thresholds.[42]

Glucose availability for cellular energy is determined by perfusion and individual glucose utilization, not only BG. Factors that impact neurologic sensitivity to lower BG values include comorbidities: neonatal sepsis, perinatal stress, shock, congenital heart disease, and respiratory illnesses; gestational age and size, and complicated persistent hypoglycemia disorders, that is, hyperinsulinism, counterregulatory hormone deficiency, gluconeogenesis disorders, and inborn errors of metabolism.[43] A continuous supply of glucose is vital for normal cellular metabolism, especially in the brain.

Appropriate treatment of NH is guided by the correct classification.[43,44] Short-term, transient NH is the most common type, occurring early in the newborn period (3–12 hours after delivery). It may be symptomatic or asymptomatic, and represents a temporary inability to maintain a normal BG concentration during transition from intrauterine to extrauterine life, and usually responds rapidly to treatment. Persistent NH is relatively rare, characterized by severe and persistent or recurrent hypoglycemia with prolonged need for high glucose infusion rates (GIR) and medications. It is often related to a primary disorder of hormone excess or enzyme deficiency, for example, hyperinsulinism, hormonal deficiencies, hereditary defects in carbohydrate, amino acid, or fatty acid metabolism. The PES provides excellent guidance for evaluation of infants with persistent hypoglycemia.[21]

Despite the ongoing debate about what constitutes clinically significant hypoglycemia, clinical practice remains primarily based on expert opinion. The controversy persists regarding whether a low BG in healthy newborns is a normal, transient phenomenon.[32] Although the safety of asymptomatic hypoglycemia is unclear, recent evidence suggests neurodevelopmental sequelae from even transient asymptomatic NH.[10,20]

NEONATAL GLUCOSE HOMEOSTASIS

After clamping of the umbilical cord, the newborn must abruptly draw on its own stored substrates until a source of carbohydrate is provided. Serum glucose levels decline in healthy term infants until approximately 1 to 3 hours of age ("nadir," or lowest point) before spontaneously increasing. The nadir is thought to be important for activating glycogenolysis, followed by gluconeogenesis. Anoxia, cord clamping, and tactile stimulation initiate the cascade of BG demand, signaling the release of epinephrine and norepinephrine and a concomitant suppression of insulin. Rising catecholamine levels stimulate the release of glucagon and lipolysis, resulting in hepatic gluconeogenesis. In concert with falling serum glucose, hepatic glycogen phosphorylase initiates glycogenolysis, resulting in hepatic glucose release.[20,21] In the preterm infant, this enzymatic process may be immature and ineffective, thus contributing to their risk for NH.[45]

Insulin serves as an important growth factor for the fetus. The BG level at which insulin continues to be secreted is significantly lower in the fetus compared with children and adults. After delivery, insulin secretion continues at the fetal rate, despite lower BG, contributing to a "transitional NH." This postnatal failure to suppress insulin secretion may be exacerbated by other factors and lead to lower BG than may be safe for the vulnerable brain, especially in at-risk infants.[20] Under normal conditions, the newborn produces glucose at a rate of 4 to 6 mg/kg/min to maintain homeostasis, twice an adult's.[44] This higher glucose production rate is likely due to the newborn's increased brain-to-body mass ratio and the brain's high-glucose requirement, thus underscoring the importance of close surveillance of BG in stressed and at-risk infants.

HYPOGLYCEMIA AND THE NEONATAL BRAIN

The brain uses glucose as its primary metabolic fuel, thus hypoglycemia can be a sign of neuronal energy deficiency. The neonatal brain continues to grow rapidly after delivery, using glucose for structural proteins and myelination.[46] During periods of low BG, the term neonatal brain was thought to use alternative fuel sources, for example, lactate, amino acids, and ketone. Although this process is not well understood, it was considered neuroprotective against brain injury.[24] However, recent findings question the availability of ketones and free fatty acids as alternative brain fuels, due to immature liver function and hormonal response/control.[20,21] Furthermore, with persistent NH and in preterm or SGA infants, these alternative fuel sources may not be available. The potential for structural brain injury from hypoglycemia is exacerbated by perinatal risk factors, for example, hypoxia, seizures, and pathologic jaundice, because alternative energy substrates may be unable to be used.[24] Ultimately, glucose is the only substrate that is protective of brain cell function, and it is reasonable to consider BG levels less than 50 mg/dL (2.2 mmol/L) as potentially neuroglycopenic.[21]

NEUROLOGIC IMPACT OF HYPOGLYCEMIA AND NEURODEVELOPMENTAL OUTCOMES

The human brain is highly vulnerable to injury when deprived of an adequate supply of glucose, especially during childhood when the brain is dynamically developing.[26] Cerebral injury following NH includes cortical neuronal injury, cerebral cortical atrophy, parenchymal hemorrhage and ischemic stroke, and white matter injury in the parietal and occipital lobes.[11,47–51] Neurologic outcomes following symptomatic hypoglycemia include intellectual disability, cerebral palsy, blindness, and epilepsy.[8,11,16,50,52–56] Infants with hypoxic-ischemic encephalopathy and hypoglycemia are at increased risk for brain injury, underscoring the importance of ensuring these infants are euglycemic.[57]

Despite the common occurrence of NH, there is a paucity of information on resultant neurodevelopmental outcomes. A systematic review on neurodevelopmental outcomes after NH in the first week of life found most studies were of poor methodologic quality, and none could validly quantify impact on neurodevelopment.[26] The knowledge gaps surrounding NH persist, including BG value that adversely affects brain function in conditions such as SGA, IDM, LPT, encephalopathy, seizures, and sepsis, along with the long-term neurologic outcomes of newborns with asymptomatic hypoglycemia.[5] The impact of transient NH and academic achievement in 10-year-old, fourth-grade students was recently reported.[6] Three BG cutoffs were analyzed: less than 35 mg/dL (1.9 mmol/L), less than 40 mg/dL (2.2 mmol/L), and less than 45 mg/dL (2.5 mmol/L). After controlling for a variety of factors, the investigators concluded that with progressively lower BG values, literacy and mathematics proficiency declined as the BG declined. This study raises concerns regarding the safety of permitting a low BG, especially in at-risk infants who may be less resilient to lower BG.

Another recent study reports on the neurodevelopmental outcomes at age 4.5 years in at-risk newborns enrolled in a dextrose-gel treatment trial (CHYLD study: Children with Hypoglycemia and Their Later Development).[10] Using a BG treatment threshold of less than 47 mg/dL (2.6 mmol/L), the investigators reported that those with NH (matched with a normoglycemic cohort) had an increased risk of poor visual motor and executive function. Executive function is an important predictor of behavior and academic achievement, including problem solving, planning, working memory, attention control and inhibition, and goal-directed behavior.[10,58]

RISK FACTORS FOR NEONATAL HYPOGLYCEMIA

Glucose homeostasis depends on a balance between glucose utilization, an adequate supply of metabolic substrates, and intact regulatory mechanisms. Risk factors for NH include both maternal and fetal/neonatal states, stressors, and diseases, with one or a combination of the following causes: (1) insufficient glycogen stores, (2) inadequate glucose production, (3) inability to synthesize glucose, (4) increased glucose utilization, and/or (5) excessive insulin production (hyperinsulinism).[44,59] **Table 1** lists the most commonly identified causes of NH; however, most causes of NH are multifactorial.

SIGNS AND SYMPTOMS OF NEONATAL HYPOGLYCEMIA

Clinical manifestations of NH are nonspecific, subtle, and widely variable (**Table 2**).[44,59] NH can be asymptomatic or so mild symptoms are virtually undetectable. Because the newborn has a limited repertoire of neurologic responses, overlap of symptoms with other conditions is common; none are specific to or diagnostic of NH, often mimicking sepsis, brain injury, drug withdrawal, metabolic derangements, and/or respiratory distress.[22,44] If clinical manifestations are present, hypoglycemia should always be ruled out.

BLOOD GLUCOSE SCREENING

The measurement of BG provides a quantification of the glucose in the bloodstream. The goal of screening is to identify abnormal levels and quickly intervene to normalize them.[19,22] Screening typically is performed by bedside "point-of-care" (POC) BG testing. POC BG screening has the advantage of rapid results at the bedside, with only a drop or 2 of blood. The whole blood devices provide good correlation to plasma glucose concentrations, averaging about 10% to 15% lower than serum values. A newer bedside POC BG test uses glucose oxidase methodology, with results paralleling plasma BG values. However, a limitation of all POC monitoring devices is their accuracy at low BG values, as the Food and Drug Administration testing standard requires accuracy only down to 20 mg/dL (1.1 mmol/L) with requirement to provide an error code for any value <10 mg/dL (0.56 mmol/L).[60] Most importantly, POC testing is only a *screening* tool: any value outside of the normal range should be confirmed

Table 1
Risk factors for neonatal hypoglycemia (detailed references available on request)

Risk Factors/Potential Causes of NH	Contributing Factors/Cause
Hyperinsulinemia	
Maternal gestational diabetes or type 2 diabetes mellitus (DM)	Especially infants of mothers with insulin requirement during pregnancy or hyperglycemia during labor, or with male infants
Maternal body mass index (BMI) >25 kg/m^2	BMI is a predictor of NH in both women with and without gestational DM, and if > 3 times the recommended amount of maternal weight gain during pregnancy
IUGR, postmaturity, placental insufficiency, birth asphyxia	Transient perinatal stress hyperinsulinemia
Birth weight >90th % (LGA)	
Hyperinsulinemic genetic conditions	ABCC8, ALDH7A1, GLUD1, HNF4A, HNF1A, HADH, UCP2, inappropriate expression of the hexokinase gene, HK1, in pancreatic β cells, mutations in the GCK gene, and recessive KATP mutations
Increased glucose utilization	
Sick or stressed infants/perinatal hypoxia-ischemia	High-energy expenditure: imbalance between hepatic output and glucose utilization, depleted glycogen stores, impaired gluconeogenesis, and increased utilization of peripheral glucose (eg, with respiratory distress)
Congenital heart disease/congestive heart disease	Cardiac glycogen quickly depleted during hypoxic events; especially if metabolic acidosis accompanies congenital heart disease
Inadequate substrate stores	
IUGR/SGA	Diminished transfer of glycogen precursors (glucose and lactate) across the placenta due to insufficiency, inadequate glycogen stores, decreased ketogenic response for gluconeogenesis
Preterm/LPT	Born before the major accumulation of glycogen, fat, and protein; immaturity of their glucose regulatory hormones and enzyme systems; LPT after maternal antenatal steroid treatment
Miscellaneous risk factors	
Maternal medications	Chlorpropamide, or benzthiazide, beta-adrenergic (eg, those used for tocolysis), propranolol (beta-blockers), sulfonylureas (used for treatment of type 2 diabetes), thiazide diuretics, tricyclic antidepressants, intrapartum glucose administration, regional anesthesia

(*continued on next page*)

Table 1
(*continued*)

Risk Factors/Potential Causes of NH	Contributing Factors/Cause
Iatrogenic causes	Malposition of umbilical artery catheters, exchange transfusion, cold stress (hypothermia)
Inborn errors of metabolism	Deficiency of enzymes for mobilization of substrates and utilization of carbohydrates, fats, or amino acids (eg, galactosemia, fructose intolerance, glycogen storage diseases, and maple syrup urine disease, carnitine deficiency, propionic acidemia) and fatty acid enzyme deficiencies
Hormonal deficiencies	Hypopituitarism, hypothyroidism, adrenal insufficiency, and growth hormone deficiency, adrenal (cortisol) deficiency
Congenital disorders	Beckwith-Wiedemann syndrome, Turner syndrome, Down syndrome, Costello syndrome, congenital hypopituitarism, congenital adrenal hyperplasia, and Sotos syndrome
Defects of glucose transporter	GLUT 1, 2, and/or 3 deficiencies
Polycythemia (IDM, IUGR, maternal chronic hypertension, maternal cigarette smoking)	Increased intrauterine erythropoiesis; increased red blood cell pool leads to increased glucose utilization

with laboratory testing of a plasma glucose concentration, but treatment should not be delayed while waiting for confirmation.[22]

Several factors can influence the accuracy of POC BG results. Polycythemia may underestimate and significant anemia may overestimate the true BG value.[44] A sample from a poorly perfused extremity may not accurately reflect the BG, therefore, warming the heel with a chemical, temperature-control heat pack will increase blood flow to the extremity and improve accuracy.[44] The first drop of blood may contain cleansing antiseptic and/or excessive interstitial fluid that may cause sample dilution or clotting.[61]

Plasma (serum) glucose levels are dependent on timely laboratory processing to prevent red blood cells from further metabolizing glucose, resulting in falsely low

Table 2
Symptoms of neonatal hypoglycemia

Central Nervous System	Respiratory System	Cardiovascular System
Jitteriness, tremors	Grunting	Tachycardia
Irritability	Tachypnea	Bradycardia
Hypothermia	Cyanosis	Cardiomegaly
Sweating	Apnea	Congestive heart failure
Lethargy/stupor		Asystole
Hypotonia		
High-pitched, weak, abnormal cry		
Feeding difficulty/poor sucking		
Seizures		
Coma		

serum glucose values. Glucose levels may decrease 15 to 20 mg/dL/h (0.8–1.1 mmol/L/h) when a blood sample stands at room temperature. Ideally BG samples should be put on ice or be collected in a red-top serum separator or a gray-top fluoride glycolytic inhibitor tube to prevent degradation of glucose levels.[62,63]

TREATMENT STRATEGIES FOR NEONATAL HYPOGLYCEMIA

Management strategies for NH are directed at: (1) screening of infants at risk, (2) treatment to normalize BG, and (3) identifying the cause of persistent hypoglycemia. However, the primary objective is to *prevent* hypoglycemia. The current standard preventative measure in otherwise healthy at-risk infants is frequent milk feedings (breast or infant formula). Glucose water feeding has been long abandoned because milk feedings provide carbohydrate (lactose) as well as protein and fat, which support gluconeogenesis. Feedings should be initiated within the first 30 to 60 minutes of life with POC screening in at-risk infants approximately 30 minutes after and before subsequent feeds.[64–66] If the prefeed POC BG is lower than the treatment threshold, a repeat test should be done 1 hour after the feed. Breastfeeding may be supplemented with up to 5 mL/kg of expressed breast milk or infant formula.[64] The recommended frequency for breastfeeding is 8 to 12 times per day in the first few days following birth. Skin-to-skin contact immediately after birth facilitates early breastfeeding and reduces energy expenditure.[67]

If the BG remains below treatment threshold despite feeding, intravenous (IV) dextrose therapy should be considered.[19] In light of the lower BG thresholds in the AAP algorithm,[19] and their focus on the first 24 hours of life, it is imperative to closely monitor infants for signs and symptoms of hypoglycemia. BG screening should be extended if POC values are borderline or unstable, as a recent study found that more than one-third of NH occurred *after* 24 hours of age.[7] Any infant who is symptomatic with a BP less than 40 mg/dL (2.2 mmol/L) should not be treated by using the algorithm and requires IV dextrose treatment.

Intravenous Dextrose

When the BG cannot be stabilized with feedings, the infant is symptomatic, ill, or early preterm, IV dextrose is indicated, with management by neonatal health care providers in a special care nursery (SCN) or neonatal intensive care unit (NICU). IV dextrose should be considered a medication with a calculated dosage, including the amount of glucose provided in a prescribed volume and the GIR. A 10% dextrose concentration means there are 10 g of dextrose per 100 mL or 100 mg/mL.

$$\frac{10\text{ g dextrose}}{100\text{ mL}} = \frac{0.1\text{ g}}{\text{mL}} = 0.1\text{ g} \times 1000 = \frac{100\text{ mg dextrose}}{\text{mL}}$$

The standard practice for NH is administration of an initial 2 mL/kg of 10% dextrose (200 mg dextrose/kg, "mini-bolus"), followed by a continuous infusion of 10% dextrose.[22] A recent study monitoring continuous interstitial glucose concentrations in newborns at risk for NH demonstrated worse neurodevelopmental outcomes when there was rapid correction of glucose.[10] Animal studies suggest that hypoglycemia followed by higher glucose concentrations can cause neuronal injury because of changes in cerebral perfusion and generation of reactive oxygen species.[68,69] It is apparent that more research is needed in this area to guide the safest rate and method for raising the BG.

Measurement of BG should occur no longer than 30 minutes after initiation of IV dextrose and then be followed closely, every 1 to 2 hours, until it stabilizes within the treatment target.[22] If the BG falls to less than target, a mini-bolus may be repeated, and the GIR increased. The PES recommends a target BG >50 mg/dL (2.8 mmol/L) at <48 hours of life and greater than 60 mg/dL (3.3 mmol/L) thereafter.[21]

The GIR is calculated using the dextrose concentration, IV rate, and the infant's weight and is dosed in milligrams per kilogram per minute.

$$\text{GIR} = \frac{\%\ \text{dextrose} \times \text{IV rate} \times 0.167}{\text{kg}} = \text{mg/kg/min}$$

Example: 3-kg infant on D10W at 10 mL/h.

$$\frac{10\%\ \text{dextrose} \times 10\ \text{mL/h} \times 0.167}{3\ \text{kg}} = 5.57\ \text{mg/kg/min}$$

The starting GIR should approximate the neonatal glucose production rate: 4 to 6 mg/kg/min.[44] Initiating IV dextrose at a lower GIR (3–5 mg/kg/min) for an IDM may prevent overstimulation of insulin secretion. Conversely, the intrauterine growth restricted (IUGR) infant, who has a greater brain/body mass ratio, increased peripheral insulin sensitivity, and transient hyperinsulinemia, may require a starting GIR of 6 to 8 mg/kg/min.[25] Placement of a central line, such as an umbilical venous catheter or percutaneously inserted central catheter, should be considered when an IV dextrose concentration greater than 12.5% is needed to provide the appropriate GIR.

MEDICATIONS FOR TREATMENT OF NEONATAL HYPOGLYCEMIA

When it is not possible to control BG with enteral feedings, standard practice has been to admit the infant to an SCN or NICU for further treatment, separating them from their mother. Emerging evidence supports treatment of NH with oral dextrose gel (DG) in the mother/baby unit, although vigilant assessment is still indicated.

Dextrose Gel: An Emerging New Therapy

Treatment of hypoglycemia using DG was first described by researchers in New Zealand and Ireland.[70,71] In 2013, the first randomized, double-blind, placebo-controlled study evaluating the use of DG versus placebo gel in at-risk, 35-week gestation and older infants was published, "The Sugar Babies Study."[72,73] Infants were randomized to receive either DG or placebo gel if BG was less than 47 mg/dL (2.6 mmol/L). Nonhypoglycemic infants received usual care and monitoring. Treatment failure was defined as a BG <47 mg/dL (2.6 mmol/L) after 2 treatment attempts. The researchers concluded that treatment with DG combined with enteral feedings was more effective in reversing NH than feedings alone. In addition to the cost saving of avoiding NICU admission, the investigator's suggested DG helped reduce maternal anxiety and improve successful breastfeeding rates.[72] Of significant concern, however, were the reports of impaired neurodevelopmental outcomes when the study children were evaluated at 4.5 years,[10] and the resulting question regarding whether asymptomatic hypoglycemia is safe for the at-risk newborn's brain.

The Sugar Babies study[72] has been cited to justify development and implementation of DG protocols in the United States.[74–76] However, these protocols advocate for lower BG treatment thresholds than used in the New Zealand study,[72,73] as well as those recommended by the PES.[21] Optimal use of DG is still under investigation,[3,32,77] and until more evidence is available on neurologic safety, clinicians are cautioned to consider strict adherence to the DG protocol and BG treatment thresholds used by the New Zealand researchers.[72,73]

Glucocorticoids

Steroids, including hydrocortisone and dexamethasone, have been used when downward titration of the GIR results in recurrent hypoglycemia.[78] Glucocorticoids reverse hypoglycemia by reducing insulin secretion and increasing insulin resistance, amplifying gluconeogenesis and glycogenolysis. Potential significant side effects (hypertension, feeding intolerance, growth suppression, and adverse neurodevelopmental outcomes) have limited the application of this therapy in treating NH.

Diazoxide

Diazoxide is frequently initiated for persistent hyperinsulinemic hypoglycemia of infancy when the BG is unable to be stabilized using IV dextrose, or a high GIR (20 mg/kg/min) cannot be weaned.[78] Diazoxide inhibits insulin secretion through stabilization of the opening of ATP-sensitive potassium channels in pancreatic beta cells.[78] Diazoxide is administered orally, with dosage ranges from 5 to 15 mg/kg/day in 2 or 3 divided doses. The dose is titrated up or down as needed to establish stable BG levels. A reported side effect of diazoxide is hypertrichosis, excessive hair growth of the eyebrows, forehead, and back, which resolves after therapy is discontinued. Sodium retention is another common side effect of diazoxide and is often treated by adding chlorothiazide to decrease fluid retention. Infants treated with diazoxide are at higher risk for developing pulmonary hypertension (PH). Therefore, infants at risk for PH (eg, meconium aspiration, respiratory distress syndrome, transient tachypnea, pneumonia, sepsis, congenital diaphragmatic hernia, or congenital heart disease) should be closely monitored (www.fda.gov/Drugs/DrugSafety/ucm454833.htm). PH should improve or resolve when diazoxide is stopped. If the infant is unresponsive to diazoxide, octreotide, a long-acting somatostatin analogue may be trialed.

SUMMARY

Despite the plethora of literature related to NH, the magic BG number for treating NH and the ideal treatment strategy are still unclear. Infants who are at risk for hypoglycemia are well elucidated, and the increased risk for hypoglycemia, when multiple risk factors are present, is also clear. Following current guidelines for practice to identify infants at greatest risk, using excellent assessment skills for identifying symptoms of NH in the at-risk newborn, optimizing breastfeeding support, and identifying situations where screening may need to be extended are essential for preventing clinically significant NH. It is hoped that future randomized trials will provide further guidance and knowledge related to NH, prevention and treatment strategies, and neurodevelopmental outcomes.

REFERENCES

1. Mehta A. Prevention and management of neonatal hypoglycaemia. Arch Dis Child Fetal Neonatal Ed 1994;70(1):F54–9 [discussion: F59–60].
2. Cornblath M, Hawdon JM, Williams AF, et al. Controversies regarding definition of neonatal hypoglycemia: suggested operational thresholds. Pediatrics 2000; 105(5):1141–5.
3. Hegarty JE, Harding JE, Crowther CA, et al. Oral dextrose gel to prevent hypoglycaemia in at-risk neonates. Cochrane Database Syst Rev 2017;(7).
4. Chandran S, Rajadurai V, Alim A, et al. Current perspectives on neonatal hypoglycemia, its management, and cerebral injury risk. Res Rep Neonatal 2015;2015(5): 17–30.

5. Hay WW Jr, Raju TN, Higgins RD, et al. Knowledge gaps and research needs for understanding and treating neonatal hypoglycemia: workshop report from Eunice Kennedy Shriver national Institute of Child Health and human development. J Pediatr 2009;155(5):612–7.
6. Kaiser JR, Bai S, Gibson N, et al. Association between transient newborn hypoglycemia and fourth-grade achievement test proficiency: a population-based study. JAMA Pediatr 2015;169(10):913–21.
7. Harris DL, Weston PJ, Harding JE. Incidence of neonatal hypoglycemia in babies identified as at risk. J Pediatr 2012;161(5):787–91.
8. Boardman JP, Wusthoff CJ, Cowan FM. Hypoglycaemia and neonatal brain injury. Arch Dis Child Educ Pract Ed 2013;98(1):2–6.
9. Lucas A, Morley R, Cole TJ. Adverse neurodevelopmental outcome of moderate neonatal hypoglycaemia. BMJ 1988;297(6659):1304–8.
10. McKinlay CJD, Alsweiler JM, Anstice NS, et al. Association of neonatal glycemia with neurodevelopmental outcomes at 4.5 years. JAMA Pediatr 2017;171(10):972–83.
11. Burns CM, Rutherford MA, Boardman JP, et al. Patterns of cerebral injury and neurodevelopmental outcomes after symptomatic neonatal hypoglycemia. Pediatrics 2008;122(1):65–74.
12. Vannucci RC, Vannucci SJ. Hypoglycemic brain injury. Semin Neonatol 2001;6(2):147–55.
13. Caraballo RH, Sakr D, Mozzi M, et al. Symptomatic occipital lobe epilepsy following neonatal hypoglycemia. Pediatr Neurol 2004;31(1):24–9.
14. Koh TH, Aynsley-Green A, Tarbit M, et al. Neural dysfunction during hypoglycaemia. Arch Dis Child 1988;63(11):1353–8.
15. Kerstjens JM, Bocca-Tjeertes IF, de Winter AF, et al. Neonatal morbidities and developmental delay in moderately preterm-born children. Pediatrics 2012;130(2):e265–72.
16. Arhan E, Ozturk Z, Serdaroglu A, et al. Neonatal hypoglycemia: a wide range of electroclinical manifestations and seizure outcomes. Eur J Paediatr Neurol 2017;21(5):738–44.
17. Yang G, Zou L-P, Wang J, et al. Neonatal hypoglycemic brain injury is a cause of infantile spasms. Exp Ther Med 2016;11(5):2066–70.
18. Harding JE, Harris DL, Hegarty JE, et al. An emerging evidence base for the management of neonatal hypoglycaemia. Early Hum Dev 2017;104:51–6.
19. Committee on Fetus and Newborn, Adamkin DH. Postnatal glucose homeostasis in late-preterm and term infants. Pediatrics 2011;127(3):575–9.
20. Stanley CA, Rozance PJ, Thornton PS, et al. Re-evaluating "transitional neonatal hypoglycemia": mechanism and implications for management. J Pediatr 2015;166(6):1520–5.e1.
21. Thornton PS, Stanley CA, De Leon DD, et al. Recommendations from the Pediatric Endocrine Society for evaluation and management of persistent hypoglycemia in neonates, infants, and children. J Pediatr 2015;167(2):238–45.
22. Karlsen KA. The S.T.A.B.L.E. program pre-transport post-resuscitation stabilization care of sick infants : guidelines for neonatal healthcare providers: learner manual. 6th edition. Park City (UT): The S.T.A.B.L.E. Program; 2013.
23. Koh TH, Eyre JA, Aynsley-Green A. Neonatal hypoglycaemia–the controversy regarding definition. Arch Dis Child 1988;63(11):1386–8.
24. Montassir H, Maegaki Y, Ogura K, et al. Associated factors in neonatal hypoglycemic brain injury. Brain Dev 2009;31(9):649–56.

25. Rozance PJ, Hay WW Jr. New approaches to management of neonatal hypoglycemia. Matern Health Neonatol Perinatol 2016;2:3.
26. Boluyt N, van Kempen A, Offringa M. Neurodevelopment after neonatal hypoglycemia: a systematic review and design of an optimal future study. Pediatrics 2006;117(6):2231–43.
27. Puchalski M, Hummel P. The reality of neonatal pain. Adv Neonatal Care 2002; 2(5):233–44 [quiz: 245–7].
28. Harris S. Hyperinsulinism and dysinsulinism. J Am Med Assoc 1924;83(10): 729–33.
29. Hartmann AF, Jaudon JC, Morton M. Hypoglycemia. J Pediatr 11(1):1–36.
30. Hawdon JM, Ward Platt MP, Aynsley-Green A. Patterns of metabolic adaptation for preterm and term infants in the first neonatal week. Arch Dis Child 1992; 67(4 Spec No):357–65.
31. Cole MD. New factors associated with the incidence of hypoglycemia: a research study. Neonatal Netw 1991;10(4):47–50.
32. McKinlay CJ, Harding JE. Revisiting transitional hypoglycemia: only time will tell. JAMA Pediatr 2015;169(10):892–4.
33. McGowan JE. Neonatal hypoglycemia. Pediatr Rev 1999;20(7):e6–15.
34. Harris DL, Weston PJ, Battin MR, et al. A survey of the management of neonatal hypoglycaemia within the Australian and New Zealand Neonatal Network. J Paediatr Child Health 2014;50(10):E55–62.
35. Screening guidelines for newborns at risk for low blood glucose. Paediatrics Child Health 2004;9(10):723–9.
36. Adamkin DH. Neonatal hypoglycemia. Semin Fetal Neonatal Med 2017;22(1): 36–41.
37. Hoseth E, Joergensen A, Ebbesen F, et al. Blood glucose levels in a population of healthy, breast fed, term infants of appropriate size for gestational age. Arch Dis Child Fetal Neonatal Ed 2000;83(2):F117–9.
38. Adamkin DH. Neonatal hypoglycemia. Curr Opin Pediatr 2016;28(2):150–5.
39. Alkalay AL, Sarnat HB, Flores-Sarnat L, et al. Population meta-analysis of low plasma glucose thresholds in full-term normal newborns. Am J Perinatol 2006; 23(2):115–9.
40. Lucas A, Morley R. Authors reply to outcome of neonatal hypoglycaemia: complete data are needed. BMJ 1999;318(7177):194.
41. Williams AF. Neonatal hypoglycaemia: clinical and legal aspects. Semin Fetal Neonatal Med 2005;10(4):363–8.
42. McKinlay CJ, Alsweiler JM, Ansell JM, et al. Neonatal glycemia and neurodevelopmental outcomes at 2 years. N Engl J Med 2015;373(16):1507–18.
43. Stanley CA, Hardy OT. Pathophysiology of hypoglycemia. In: Polin RA, Fox WW, Abman SH, editors. Fetal and neonatal physiology. 4th edition. Philadelphia: Saunders: Elsevier; 2011. p. 568–75.
44. Devaskar SU, Garg M. Disorders of carbohydrate metabolism in the neonate. In: Martin RJ, Fanaroff AA, Walsh MC, editors. Fanaroff and Martin's neonatal-perinatal medicine: diseases of the fetus and infant, vol. 2, 10th edition. Philadelphia: Elsevier Sanders; 2015. p. 1434–59.
45. Ward Platt M, Deshpande S. Metabolic adaptation at birth. Semin Fetal Neonatal Med 2005;10(4):341–50.
46. Knickmeyer RC, Gouttard S, Kang C, et al. A structural MRI study of human brain development from birth to 2 years. J Neurosci 2008;28(47):12176–82.
47. Aslan Y, Dinc H. MR findings of neonatal hypoglycemia. AJNR Am J Neuroradiol 1997;18(5):994–6.

48. Barkovich AJ, Ali FA, Rowley HA, et al. Imaging patterns of neonatal hypoglycemia. AJNR Am J Neuroradiol 1998;19(3):523–8.
49. Murakami Y, Yamashita Y, Matsuishi T, et al. Cranial MRI of neurologically impaired children suffering from neonatal hypoglycaemia. Pediatr Radiol 1999; 29(1):23–7.
50. Filan PM, Inder TE, Cameron FJ, et al. Neonatal hypoglycemia and occipital cerebral injury. J Pediatr 2006;148(4):552–5.
51. Yalnizoglu D, Haliloglu G, Turanli G, et al. Neurologic outcome in patients with MRI pattern of damage typical for neonatal hypoglycemia. Brain Dev 2007; 29(5):285–92.
52. Menni F, de Lonlay P, Sevin C, et al. Neurologic outcomes of 90 neonates and infants with persistent hyperinsulinemic hypoglycemia. Pediatrics 2001;107(3): 476–9.
53. Udani V, Munot P, Ursekar M, et al. Neonatal hypoglycemic brain - injury a common cause of infantile onset remote symptomatic epilepsy. Indian Pediatr 2009; 46(2):127–32.
54. Montassir H, Maegaki Y, Ohno K, et al. Long term prognosis of symptomatic occipital lobe epilepsy secondary to neonatal hypoglycemia. Epilepsy Res 2010; 88(2–3):93–9.
55. Tam EW, Widjaja E, Blaser SI, et al. Occipital lobe injury and cortical visual outcomes after neonatal hypoglycemia. Pediatrics 2008;122(3):507–12.
56. Karimzadeh P, Tabarestani S, Ghofrani M. Hypoglycemia-occipital syndrome: a specific neurologic syndrome following neonatal hypoglycemia? J Child Neurol 2011;26(2):152–9.
57. Tam EW, Haeusslein LA, Bonifacio SL, et al. Hypoglycemia is associated with increased risk for brain injury and adverse neurodevelopmental outcome in neonates at risk for encephalopathy. J Pediatr 2012;161(1):88–93.
58. Ansell JM, Wouldes TA, Harding JE, et al. Executive function assessment in New Zealand 2-year olds born at risk of neonatal hypoglycemia. PLoS One 2017; 12(11):e0188158.
59. Blackburn S. Maternal, fetal, & neonatal physiology: a clinical perspective. 3rd edition. Philadephia: Elsevier Sanders; 2013.
60. U.S. Department of Health and Human Services Food and Drug Administration Center for Devices and Radiological Health Office of In Vitro Diagnostics and Radiological Health Division of Chemistry and Toxicology Devices. Blood glucose monitoring test systems for prescription point-of-care use: guidance for industry and food and drug administration staff October 11, 2016. 2016. 1755.
61. Folk LA. Guide to capillary heelstick blood sampling in infants. Adv Neonatal Care 2007;7(4):171–8.
62. Chan AY, Swaminathan R, Cockram CS. Effectiveness of sodium fluoride as a preservative of glucose in blood. Clin Chem 1989;35(2):315–7.
63. Mikesh LM, Bruns DE. Stabilization of glucose in blood specimens: mechanism of delay in fluoride inhibition of glycolysis. Clin Chem 2008;54(5):930–2.
64. Wight N, Marinelli KA. ABM clinical protocol #1: guidelines for blood glucose monitoring and treatment of hypoglycemia in term and late-preterm neonates, revised 2014. Breastfeed Med 2014;9(4):173–9.
65. Harris DL, Gamble GD, Weston PJ, et al. What happens to blood glucose concentrations after oral treatment for neonatal hypoglycemia? J Pediatr 2017;190: 136–41.
66. Cordero L, Ramesh S, Hillier K, et al. Early feeding and neonatal hypoglycemia in infants of diabetic mothers. SAGE Open Med 2013;1. 2050312113516613.

67. Lau Y, Tha PH, Ho-Lim SST, et al. An analysis of the effects of intrapartum factors, neonatal characteristics, and skin-to-skin contact on early breastfeeding initiation. Matern Child Nutr 2018;14(1).
68. Pryds O, Christensen NJ, Friis-Hansen B. Increased cerebral blood flow and plasma epinephrine in hypoglycemic, preterm neonates. Pediatrics 1990;85(2): 172–6.
69. Ennis K, Dotterman H, Stein A, et al. Hyperglycemia accentuates and ketonemia attenuates hypoglycemia-induced neuronal injury in the developing rat brain. Pediatr Res 2015;77(1–1):84–90.
70. Bourchier D, Weston P, Heron P. Hypostop for neonatal hypoglycaemia. N Z Med J 1992;105(926):22.
71. Troughton KEV, Corrigan NP, Tait RME. Hypostop gel in the treatment of neonatal hypoglycaemia: a randomised controlled trial. Arch Dis Child 2000;82(Suppl 1): A30.
72. Harris DL, Weston PJ, Signal M, et al. Dextrose gel for neonatal hypoglycaemia (the Sugar Babies Study): a randomised, double-blind, placebo-controlled trial. Lancet 2013;382(9910):2077–83.
73. Panel ODGtTNHCPG. Oral dextrose gel to treat neonatal hypoglycaemia: New Zealand clinical practice guidelines 2015. Auckland (New Zealand): Department of Paediatrics: Child and Youth Health, University of Auckland; 2015.
74. Bennett C, Fagan E, Chaharbakhshi E, et al. Implementing a protocol using glucose gel to treat neonatal hypoglycemia. Nurs Womens Health 2016;20(1): 64–74.
75. Rawat M, Chandrasekharan P, Turkovich S, et al. Oral dextrose gel reduces the need for intravenous dextrose therapy in neonatal Hypoglycemia. Biomed Hub 2016;1(3) [pii:448511].
76. Smith P. Dextrose gel for treatment of neonatal hypoglycemia. In: Iowa's statewide perinatal care program. vol. XXXII, No 1. Iowa City (IA). 2016.
77. Harding JE, Hegarty JE, Crowther CA, et al. Randomised trial of neonatal hypoglycaemia prevention with oral dextrose gel (hPOD): study protocol. BMC Pediatr 2015;15:120.
78. Sweet CB, Grayson S, Polak M. Management strategies for neonatal hypoglycemia. J Pediatr Pharmacol Ther 2013;18(3):199–208.

Big Data in Neonatal Health Care: Big Reach, Big Reward?

Lynn E. Bayne, PhD, APRN, NNP-BC[a,b,*]

KEYWORDS

- Big data • Electronic health record (EHR) • Neonatology • Cost-savings
- Clinical decision making • Healthcare analytics

KEY POINTS

- Analog-to-digital data conversion has created massive amounts of historical and real-time health care data.
- Costs associated with neonatal health issues are high.
- Big data use in the neonatal intensive care unit has the potential to facilitate earlier detection of clinical deterioration, expedite application of efficient clinical decision-making algorithms based on real-time and historical data mining, and yield significant cost-savings.

INTRODUCTION

US health care costs are high, nearly double as a percentage of the US economy, compared with other advanced, industrialized countries.[1] In 2016, $3.3 trillion, or 17.9% of the US economy, was devoted to health care, a 4.3% increase over 2015 spending. Per capita spending increased $354 to $10,348 per individual.[2] Health care has the potential to bankrupt this nation if cost containment strategies cannot be identified. Use of health care analytics and use of big data may provide a partial solution. The purpose of this review is to inform critical care nurses about the scope of health care costs and to explore a more intelligent use of data, including the viability of big data, as one opportunity to mitigate rising costs.

As recently as 1980, American health care spending was much closer to that of peer nations, as shown in **Fig. 1**.[1] What has happened to alter historic patterns in this untenable manner? Experts suggest that the disparate price tags are not because US citizens have better facilities or equipment, nor is it because US citizens have better or more access, higher service utilization rates, or better outcomes. The reason for higher costs appears to be explained by the fact that health care simply costs more in the US compared with other nations.[3,4] Health care costs in 2016 grew 1.5% faster than the nation's gross domestic product, which increased by 2.8%.[2]

Disclosure: The author has nothing to disclose.

[a] Christiana Care Health System, 4755 Ogletown-Stanton Road, Newark, DE 19716, USA; [b] Alfred I. duPont Hospital for Children, 1600 Rockland Road, Wilmington, DE 19803, USA
* Christiana Care Health System, 4755 Ogletown-Stanton Road, Newark, DE 19716.
E-mail address: LBayne@christianacare.org

Crit Care Nurs Clin N Am 30 (2018) 481–497
https://doi.org/10.1016/j.cnc.2018.07.005
ccnursing.theclinics.com
0899-5885/18/

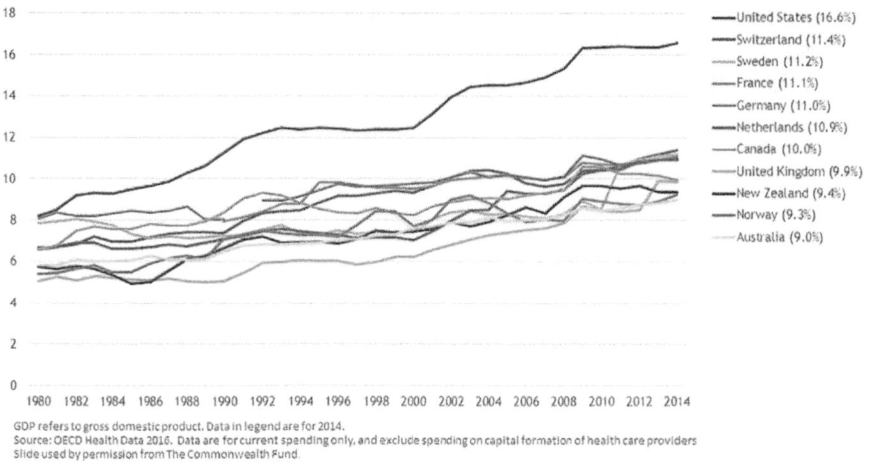

Fig. 1. Health care spending as a percentage of gross domestic product, 1980 to 2014. (*From* Schneider EC, Sarnak DO, Squires D, et al. Mirror, mirror: how the U.S. health care system compares internationally at a time of radical change. The Commonwealth Fund. Available at: https://www.commonwealthfund.org/publications/fund-reports/2017/jul/mirror-mirror-2017-international-comparison-reflects-flaws-and. Accessed February 12, 2018; with permission.)

Just as alarming is that sources project that total health care spending from both public and private sources is expected to increase to almost 20% of the economy by 2025 (**Fig. 2**).[5,6] Proponents of the Affordable Care Act (ACA), the most substantial health policy reform in the history of the nation, were hopeful that this legislation would provide a pathway to solving the fiscal problem. Conceptually, the legislation was planned to take a preventative, community-based approach to disease—but still, the costs are rising. ACA critics have challenged that the legislation has not

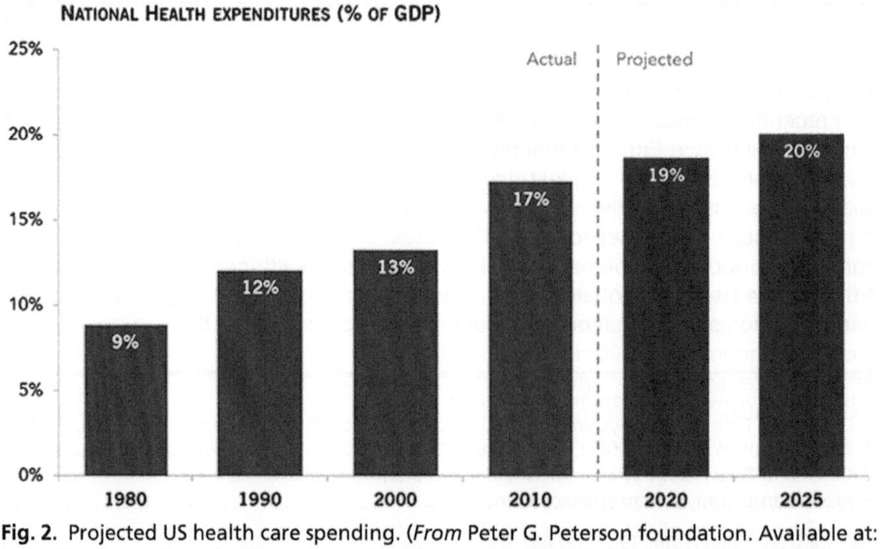

Fig. 2. Projected US health care spending. (*From* Peter G. Peterson foundation. Available at: https://www.pgpf.org/finding-solutions/healthcare. Accessed December 16, 2017; with permission.)

gone far enough to contain health care costs or improve quality of care with better outcomes.[7]

One of the ACA cornerstones is a requirement for digitization of patient information and adoption of electronic health records (EHR) in the community and hospital settings, accessible by patients or their families, when the patient is a minor. This requirement was, and continues to be, a daunting task. Health care has historically generated massive amounts of analog, hard copy data, driven by mandatory record keeping, as well as regulatory and compliance requirements.[8] Until recently, most of this data existed in paper format, making it difficult to subject clinical information to large scale processing and synthesis for the purposes of clinical decision support. With the advent of the information age that started in the 1970s with the introduction of the personal computer and software technology, it became possible to transfer analog information freely and quickly to digital format. This transition makes health care data eligible for big data analysis strategies.[9]

BIG DATA

What Is Big Data?

Big data refers to data sets so voluminous and complex that traditional data processing hardware and application software are inadequate to deal with it. Big data sets are challenged by data capture, storage, analysis, searchability, ease of sharing, ease of transfer, visualization, querying, and privacy.[10,11] If this seems like a nebulous concept despite its rising use, that is because it is. It is little more than a broad word for smashing 2 of more data sets together to generate information unavailable from a single source and then looking for a meaningful pattern. Big data was originally characterized by 3 dimensions, known as the Three V's: volume, variety, and velocity. Veracity has been added as a fourth quality because the volume of data continues to grow, and analytics matures as a science.[8,9]

Fig. 3 helps to illustrate how these concepts are linked. Big data includes information being created by machines as well as people. Volume always seems to head the list in discussions about big data and analytics. It generally refers to data sets that exceed volumes of a terabyte and beyond. Variety refers to different formats of data, as in unstructured, semi-structured, or structured. It exists in analog or digital state, but for analytical purposes, it must be converted to digital format. Velocity aptly describes the third characteristics. Data are being created extremely fast, a process which never stops, even while we sleep. It may flow, or move, in near-time or real-time; it may flow in batches or streams. The data must be captured, stored, and analyzed to be able to facilitate decision making. Veracity refers to the quality, accuracy, relevance, meaningfulness, and predictive value of data as it is produced, captured, stored, and analyzed. Data quality issues are of acute concern in health care because life or death decisions depend on accurate information. In addition, the quality of health care data, especially unstructured data, is highly variable, and all too often incorrect. Key examples of this are appreciated when one considers medical errors due to illegibly written orders or incorrectly executed verbal orders. To execute reliable clinical decision-making algorithms, the accuracy of the data is pivotal to optimal patient outcomes.[8]

Big data applications have been used in many areas: in government to understand election campaign strategies, in retail to understand consumer buying habits, in finance to calculate credit scores and credit risk, in science to understand the implications of genetics/genomics in pharmaceutical research, and in sports to improve athletic training and performance. The rhetorical question to be considered is do

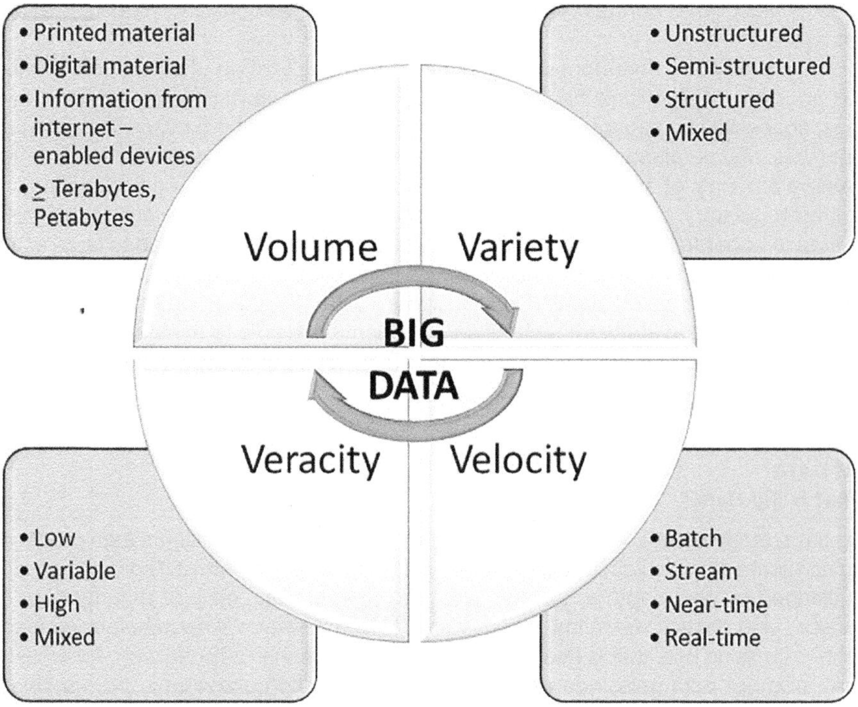

Fig. 3. The 4 V's of big data.

industries like these guarantee similar results in health care that will yield cost reduction, improved efficiency, and enhanced clinical decision support and offer better, safer patient outcomes?

Why Is It Time for Big Data Health Care Analytics Now?

As big data health care analytics takes root, it will likely refer less to the data set size and more to the descriptive, predictive, or prescriptive dimensions of analytics that extract value from patterns and other meaningful information collected from a multitude of patient data sources (**Table 1**). Descriptive analytics are where most organizations start. Most health care data, including clinical documentation, claims data, patient surveys, or diagnostic testing, tell clinicians what has already happened. Although this information is a good place to start, and can be valuable for clinical or operational management, there is only so much that can be gleaned from a historical record. Predictive analytics is the ability to extrapolate the course of future events from the descriptive data. It requires large volumes of near- or real-time data that can be subjected to nontraditional analyses. The patterns within the data are generally not revealed by traditional statistical methods, nor are their linkages to other important factors easily identifiable.[8,12,13]

Computers are ubiquitous at the bedside through charting systems that provide the foundation of the EHR, as well as through the cadre of devices used for patient care. These devices collect massive quantities of digital data and require significant storage capabilities. Furthermore, the ability to process and synthesize all this health care data cannot keep up with the rate of data production. These factors present important challenges, which must be solved for data scientists to fulfill the promise of supporting a

Table 1
Potential sources of big data in health care

Data Source[a]	Volume	Variety	Velocity	Veracity
Clinicians' free text notes	Terabytes of stored text	Unstructured	Batch	Low, variable, high, mixed
Clinical orders (pharmacy & nonpharmacy)	Terabytes of stored text	Unstructured	Batch	Low, variable, high, mixed
Patient-generated biometric data (eg, point-of-care glucose)	Few patients at first, but will grow	Structured	Batch, near-time	High
Wearable personal health care devices	Few patients at first, but will grow	Structured	Batch, near-time	High
Physiologic monitoring data	Very large with high resolution	Structured	Batch, near-time, real-time	High
Medical devices	Few patients at first, but will grow	Structured	Batch, near-time, real-time	High
Medical imaging	Petabytes	Unstructured, structured	Batch, near-time, real-time	High
Laboratory data	Very large across all patients	Structured	Batch	High
Genomics	~100 GB per patient	Structured, standard formulas exist	Batch	High
Credit card & purchasing data	Very large across all patients	Unstructured, semi-structured, structured	Batch	Low, variable, high, mixed
Social media data (eg, Facebook, Blogs, Web sites)	Very large across all patients	Unstructured, semi-structured, structured	Batch	Low, variable, high, mixed
Smartphones	Very large across all patients	Unstructured, semi-structured, structured	Batch, near-time, real-time	Low, variable, high, mixed
Insurance claims	Terabytes of stored text	Unstructured, semi-structured, structured	Batch	Low, variable, high, mixed
Billing	Terabytes of stored text	Unstructured, semi-structured, structured	Batch	Low, variable, high, mixed
Other administrative data (eg, patient survey, safety reports)	Terabytes of stored text	Unstructured, semi-structured, structured	Batch	Low, variable, high, mixed

[a] Based on conversion of patient health record and associated data having been converted from analog to digital format, a critical step for health care analytics to be applied.

wide range of health care functions, including targeted, diagnosis-specific clinical decision support offered in a more timely, cost-efficient manner. When operational, any patient's data will not be treated in isolation. It will be compared alongside thousands of other historic and current patients, highlighting specific threats and patterns that emerge during the comparisons. Descriptive analytical techniques will play an important role in the development of this pathway. Furthermore, this capability potentially facilitates consideration of sophisticated, individualized treatment algorithms backed up by data from other patients with the same condition, genetic factors, socioeconomic status, and lifestyle based on prescriptive analytics. Population health management targeting prevention should become a reality if experts are able to harness the power of mobile devices coupled with wearable personal data trackers to prevent illness before it occurs. Meeting this goal will involve aggressive use of predictive and prescriptive analytical techniques. In both targeted-treatment and population health management, the financial returns on investment and improved outcomes should have the positive influence of U.S health care containment that has not been realized since 1980.[8,12,13]

Challenges of Big Data Use in Health Care

Big data use in health care seems overwhelming due to its sheer volume, its diversity, the speed with which it must be managed, and the reliability that it must offer to inform clinical decision making. As previously suggested in this review, the volume of stored data grows exponentially year on year due to the transition from analog-to-digital data format, all made possible by the computer. Experts state that 90% of all data has been generated within the last 2 years of any rolling retrospective 2-year epoch. Eighty percent of data exists in unstructured format, compared with 20% existing in structured format.[8] **Table 2** gives some typical examples of data volume to provide clarity for possible challenges that lay ahead as this science grows in maturity. By 2011, the volume of US health care had reached 150 exabytes (10^{18} gigabytes, GB). As this accumulation trend continues, big data accumulated by US health care has reached the zettabyte (10^{21} GB) threshold and is expected to be rapidly followed by the yottabyte (10^{24} GB) milestone.[8,14] The brontobyte will be part of the future of health care analytics to enable capture and storage of sensor data. Data set storage will become even more challenged and may become subject to data silos so that their patterns become difficult from which to extract insights. An example of this problem occurs when the hospital-based EHR cannot communicate effectively with the community-based EHR. It also creates significant challenges in data sharing with the global health community.

Implications of Big Data in Neonatal Health Care

Final 2016 birth data reported 3,945,875 live births in the United States, down 1% from 2015.[15] Preterm births (<37 weeks) increased from 9.63% to 9.85%, compared with 2015 data, a 20% increase. Most of the increase was among infants born late preterm. An increase in the percentage of low-birth-weight infants (<2500 g) from 8.07% to 8.17% was also reported in a slow, upward trend that has continued from 2012 data.[16]

Research also suggests that it is likely that US neonatal intensive care units (NICUs) are seeing more admissions than ever. Is it because mothers are less healthy than in the past or is it because illness detection methods are improving, or is it something else? Data published in 2015 used time trend analysis to describe NICU admission rates for US newborns across the continuum of gestational age and birth weight. Overall, admission rates during the 6-year period from 2007 to 2012 increased from 64.0 to 77.9 per 1000 live births.[17] If 2016 NICU admission rates mirror patterns from this citation, it suggests that approximately 307,383 US babies were admitted for higher-level

Table 2
Quantifying big data volume in health care

Data Volume[a]	Storage Volume	Clinical Example
Byte	8 bits	A single character in the EHR
Kilobyte (10^3)	1000 bytes	½ page, typed
Megabyte (10^6)	1000 kilobytes	A small digital photograph
Gigabyte (10^9)	1000 megabytes	A pick-up truck filled with printed pages from the EHR
Terabyte (10^{12})	1000 gigabytes	Most new hard drives on a bedside computer on wheels have at least 1 TB; 500 TB of new data per day are ingested in Facebook databases
Petabyte (10^{15})	1000 terabytes	All radiographs digitized in a large hospital system
Exabytes (10^{18})[b]	1000 petabytes	250 million DVDs filled with patient data; 1 EB of data is created on the Internet each day
Zettabyte (10^{21})[c]	1000 exabytes	Global digital data are expected to reach 44 zettabytes by 2020
Yottabyte (10^{24})	1000 zettabytes	250 trillion DVDs filled with patient data
Brontobyte (10^{27})	1000 yottabytes	Our digital tomorrow in health care; likely to be the measurement necessary

[a] Table based on conversion of analog data from patient has been converted to digital format, a critical step for healthcare analytics to be applied.
[b] Healthcare passed Exabyte threshold in 2011.
[c] Humanity passed Zettabyte threshold in 2010.

special or intensive care. It also means that the economic burden of NICU care is and continues to be an important contributor to US health care spending, partially accounting for rising costs.[18]

An examination of overall US health care costs suggests that 5% of patients in any given care area accounts for 50% of the spending in that care area. To embellish on a previous reference, one approach to reducing health care costs from the 2025 estimates is to identify the high-cost patients in an identified specialty and manage them more effectively. This case management approach has met with varying success in health care settings. In the adult world, patients diagnosed with asthma, high cholesterol, hypertension, cancer, chronic obstructive pulmonary disease, heart disease, and stroke have the highest per capita spending.[5,19]

In the NICU, it follows that extremely low-gestational-age newborns are among the highest economic consumers of NICU dollars, mainly due to illness acuity, and overall length of stay. Common complications, such as sepsis, intraventricular hemorrhage, periventricular leukomalacia, necrotizing enterocolitis, retinopathy of prematurity, and an assortment of respiratory conditions that evolve into bronchopulmonary dysplasia, can all add to the cost of care beyond the primary diagnosis. Babies with hypoxic-ischemic encephalopathy (HIE), congenital birth defects, genetic abnormalities, and/or those that require extracorporeal membrane oxygenation may also fall into the 5% of newborns who consume a large amount of newborn health care expenses.[20–22] Case management in the NICU dates to 1992.[23–25] As in the adult world, the effectiveness of this cost-containment strategy has met with varying success. Despite identification of high-risk neonatal patients, costs on these special newborns has not consistently yielded substantial cost reductions and/or outcomes improvement. Hence, it is time to look for other solutions, that is, where big data in neonatal health care as part of the overall health care analytics strategy may be a timely solution. It holds promise to yield real-time clinical decision-making, data-driven algorithms from massive historic and real-time databases, and to offer the greatest potential for NICU cost-savings and neonatal outcome improvement. To be successful though, several issues must be considered for big data analytics to be incorporated into neonatal health care. Five issues are proposed in **Table 3**. Although considering these issues, construction of robust, personalized, and impactful neonatal algorithms, 4 general areas require intensive focus within the neonatal health care analytics framework: prevention, triage, decompensation, and readmission.

Table 3
Issues influencing effective implementation of big data analytics in neonatal health care

	Issue
1	What approach should be taken to identify high-risk obstetric and NICU patients?
2	What measurements sources can be incorporated to improve predictions? • Racial • Socioeconomic status • Parental marital status • Parental mental health status • Others
3	How can clinicians identify which patients are most likely to benefit from an intervention and what specific interventions are likely to yield the greatest improvement in care?
4	Does the algorithm or model have sufficient representation from the target group and/or population of interest?
5	Are guidelines and/or algorithms capable of dynamic changes and ability to customize or tailor intervention to the individual patient?

Prevention

Attention to prevention means neonatal data analytical scientists must possess imagination and a dare-to-dream mindset. What if some of those approximate 307,383 post-delivery NICU admissions could safely be avoided? In an ideal world, the causes for preterm delivery could be identified through a synthesis of socioeconomic data, genomic research, obstetric and medical risk factors, intermittent physical examinations, and ultrasounds. When coupled with wearable personal devices (some still not developed) and mobile technology, an early warning system channeled to the mother and her caregiver or caregivers in a real-time format becomes a plausible theoretic solution. The goal of term pregnancy for every pregnant woman becomes less idealistic.[8]

Triage

Triage begins before delivery for all fetuses. Every laboring mother is assessed before delivery for estimating her newborn's potential of risk complications. Triage is used for several reasons, such as managing staff and bed resources, anticipating the need for specialized personnel at delivery, and the overall strategy for managing the fetal transition to extrauterine life. The APGAR score was developed in 1952.[26] It represents an early example of neonatal big data use (and misuse) in a descriptive analytics approach. Five proxies of stability were identified by Dr Virginia Apgar, an anesthesiologist. The primary intent of assigning the score 0, 1, or 2 to each parameter was to determine the impact of maternal anesthesia on the newborn, a time when it was common to use more anesthesia during childbirth compared with current practices in the last 2 to 3 decades. Five areas constitute the mnemonic APGAR: *a*ctivity (muscle tone), *p* (pulse), *g*rimace (reflex irritability), *a*ppearance (color), and *r*espiration (work of breathing). A challenge of this tool is that there is significant interrater variability in its application, with 3 of the parameters being subjective.[26,27] Furthermore, some researchers extended the tool's utility beyond Dr Apgar's original intent. Nevertheless, publications have attempted to correlate APGAR scores with various neurodevelopmental outcomes. The legal community gravitated to these findings and has used APGAR as a surrogate for proposed ineffective resuscitation, with possible causation of perinatal asphyxia, now more appropriately referred to as HIE.[28] Data show that up to 840,000 (23%) of all neonatal deaths worldwide, may be due to HIE.[29] Although APGAR may be *a* factor that should be considered in development of big data-generated clinical decision-making algorithms for HIE management, it should not be *the* factor in management or outcome prediction. Imagine an era of modern big data triage techniques whereby the index patient (ie, the baby about to be born) and his or her fetal heart rate and fetal heart rate variability, in combination with physiologic parameters, such as APGAR score, cord pH, SARNAT score, and real-time index patient responses to resuscitation interventions, are compared with a massive neonatal database, driving the generation of an individualized plan of care to guide an efficient, cost-effective clinical treatment plan on admission to the NICU. It seems likely that unnecessary tests could be better avoided, and length of stay could be optimized. Just as important, legal costs related to unsubstantiated use of APGAR scores as they relate to HIE may be an important factor in unbalanced health care costs compared with other nations. Nevertheless, legal costs as they related to US health care expenses cannot be overlooked. Data from 2008 suggest that this financial burden is 2.4% of the total health care expenditure.[30]

An apparently successful example of big data synthesis is changing triage management of newborns at risk for early-onset sepsis (EOS) based on multivariate predictive analytical modeling for infants born at $\geq$34 weeks' gestation. Using an interactive, online EOS calculator in conjunction with a specific clinical decision-making algorithm, a significant reduction in US NICU admissions is being realized. In this era of antibiotic stewardship, the goal of this hallmark work is to reduce unnecessary newborn exposure to antibiotics, thought to be an important factor in the origins of drug resistance.[31]

Historically, it is estimated that thousands of US newborns are evaluated for possible EOS each year. To reduce the risk of antibiotic exposure, researchers analyzed historical data from 14 California and Massachusetts hospitals, conducting a multicenter 2-step analysis of 608,014 births ≥34 weeks. In step 1, discriminant analysis techniques showed that use of 3 continuous variables and 2 categorical variables available in the immediate perinatal period yield a reliable preliminary antenatal probability of neonatal bacterial EOS among newborns (**Table 4**). In step 2, a simplified set of quantitative and qualitative clinical findings detectable through laboratory data neonatal physical examination are combined with the maternal data retrieved in step 1, to yield a new posterior risk probability. This information can be used real-time by clinicians to guide treatment decisions and more judicious use of antibiotics.

Efficacy of this predictive algorithmic modeling has since been proven in an observational study conducted over 6 years on 204,485 neonates born at 35 weeks' gestation within the 14 study hospitals in the Kaiser Permanente Integrated Health Care System. Specifically, the findings show that a combination of these 2 steps based on analysis of historical big data, combined with a real-time data calculator, ideally located in the EHR or in a caregiver's mobile device can result in substantial savings, in addition to antibiotic stewardship. Estimates suggest that up to 240,000 fewer US newborns will be subjected to unnecessary antibiotics each year.[31–35] If a typical 2-day stay for possible EOS is averted, the cost savings is significant. This conjecture is based on NICU cost data, as reported by one major health system, at $7250 to $8935 per day.[36] Just as important is that disruption of the mother-baby dyad is prevented, and protection of optimal breastfeeding opportunities is promoted.

Decompensation

Decompensation should receive attention in a manner like prevention and triage in the promise of a big data world. Decompensation is defined as a "loss of physiologic function or physiologic compensation; especially of the heart to maintain adequate circulation."[37] It seems likely that health care costs are directly tied to illness acuity, which is linked to overall stability. Before frank instability is apparent, analytical data scientists maintain there is likely a prodromal period and/or pattern in which multisource physiologic data could be explored to determine whether the newborn is at risk for instability and

Table 4
Early-onset sepsis variables

	Variable
Continuous	Gestational age (weeks, days) Peak maternal temperature (Celsius or Fahrenheit) Duration of amniotic membranes rupture (to nearest tenth of hour)
Categorical	Group B streptococcus status (negative, positive, unknown) Intrapartum antibiotic timing • Broad spectrum antibiotics ≥4 h before birth • Broad spectrum antibiotics 2–3.9 h before birth • Group B streptococcus-specific antibiotics ≥2 h before birth • None or any antibiotics <2 h before birth

From Kaiser Permanente. Neonatal early-onset sepsis calculator. Available at: https://neonatalsepsiscalculator.kaiserpermanente.org/InfectionProbabilityCalculator.aspx. Accessed February 6, 2018; with permission.

decompensation. Identification of the markers or patterns would allow development and deployment of an early warning system to gain the attention of frontline providers before the incident. In support of decompensation patterning, neonatal researchers have demonstrated that precursors can be identified using heart rate variability in late onset sepsis, transcutaneous carbon dioxide pattern slopes in pneumothorax, fluctuations in arterial carbon dioxide measurements in severe intraventricular hemorrhage, and cumulative exposure to hypocarbia or hypercarbia in periventricular leukomalacia.[38–43]

Readmission

Readmission marks the final area that should be considered in neonatal big data analytics. Common diagnoses that may result in readmission of neonates include jaundice, dehydration, feeding difficulties, temperature instability, infection, hypoglycemia, and respiratory difficulties, including exacerbation of bronchopulmonary dysplasia, or contraction of rhinovirus/enterovirus or respiratory syncytial virus. In some of these cases, enhanced readiness for discharge may help to prevent return to hospital. Even though there are more than 1500 NICUs with more than 20,000 beds in the United States, any readmission may stretch bed capacity as well as human resources in addition to raising costs.[44] Big data patterns may facilitate readiness for discharge through predictive analytical techniques as the state of the science matures.

Nursing Implications: How Close Are We to Big Data in Neonatal Health Care?

Practical reality is modern neonatal care is that the sick newborns are surrounded by equipment. These devices provide the source of much of the data that are needed for big data analytics. Included among this cadre of equipment are cardiorespiratory monitors with integrated arterial and/or venous blood pressure measurement, mechanical ventilators, pulse oximetry monitors, transcutaneous carbon dioxide monitors, ECMO circuits, and smart infusion pumps. Right now, there is no easy way for the devices to communicate with each other or with the EHR. Furthermore, traditional EHR charting procedures limit a richer understanding of detailed information. Some experts maintain that important high-fidelity data are “left on the table” that could be used to inform patient care. For example, a newborn’s heart typically beats 140 times per minute, or 8400 times per hour. Depending on when and how the frontline clinician auscultates or observes the baby’s monitor, different values could be documented into the EHR. Most commercially available EHR vendors facilitate capture just one value per hour as a surrogate for an entire hour of clinical information. Practical instincts may guide the clinician’s approach to the data entry decision. Generally, it is a “top-of-the-hour” or “with-cares” assessment value. This pathway tends to yield a qualitative, underinformed discussion of clinical status during bedside rounding due to the lack of tools and techniques to analyze the complex, high-volume physiologic data stream the baby is generating.[45] So what information might be missed through the inability to use the real-time data stream to identify new patterns? Just how much data are not being put to use with current state-of-care strategies?

Data generated by NICU medical devices present both opportunities and challenges. In current practices, the devices generally do not communicate with each other, nor are they transmitting the data to any type of central repository that would allow for application of analytics. Some experts contend that this advance is closer than ever. Much in the way that smartphones and intelligent appliances have become part of everyday life, it is possible that medical devices will soon be part of the NICU “Internet of Things,” communicating with each other, yet generating massive quantities of high-volume, high-velocity, high-variety, and high-veracity data, capable of being transmitted to a theoretic central repository (**Table 5**).[45,46]

Table 5
Potential volume of big data generated from equipment surrounding a single neonatal intensive care unit patient

Data Source	Typical Sampling Rate	Number of Data Readings/Day/Device	Volume Data Acquired/Day (MB)
Two-channel electrocardiogram	1000 readings/s to generate waveform	86.4 million readings/d	500
Chest wall respiratory impedance waveform	62.5 readings/s	5.4 million readings/d	50
Mechanical ventilator/plethysmography	62.5 readings/s	5.4 million readings/d	50
End-tidal CO_2	62.5 readings/s	5.4 million readings/d	50
Heart rate	1 reading/s	86,400 readings/d	5
Respiratory rate	1 reading/s	86,400 readings/d	5
Pulse oximetry (SpO_2)	1 reading/s	86,400 readings/d	5
Arterial blood pressure via inserted catheter (mean, systolic, diastolic)	1 reading/s $\times$ 3 parameters	259,200 readings/d	15
Central venous pressure	1 reading/s	86,400 readings/d	5
Smart pump	60 readings/10 s	518,400 readings/d	30
Feeding pump	60 readings/10 s	518,400 readings/d	30
Total	Size of raw data		$\simeq$730 MB/d/patient

From McGregor C. Big data in the neonatal intensive care unit. Computer 2013;46(6):54–9; with permission.

The potential data volume alone, capable of being generated by a single critically ill newborn, is not insignificant. Approximately 730 MB data/day/baby has been measured through the Artemis Project. If one included data from the infant's microenvironment, such as an incubator, a transcutaneous CO_2 monitor, or an electroencephalogram that might be needed in cases of HIE, then it is not impossible to foresee that a single baby could generate 1 GB of data via the devices needed to sustain life and promote health.[46] As neonatal health care analytics evolves, data scientists could mine that second-by-second data to provide real-time actionable EWS information to modify a newborn's day-to-day care with the goal of protecting and/or promoting stability.

Pioneering work aimed at development of a system that can analyze both real-time and retrospective physiologic data from multiple data streams and sources, at the rate the data are generated across multiple channels, clinical conditions, diseases, and newborns cared for in multiple locations is currently underway. Cloud technology has partially solved some of the limitations that have challenged the analytical infrastructure and real-time clinical decision making.[45,46] The Artemis Project, named after the Greek goddess of childbearing, was first deployed in the NICU at The Hospital for Sick Children in August 2009. Under the guidance of Dr Carolyn McGregor, and in collaboration with the University of Ontario's Institute of Technology and IBM Canada, important research work shows great promise for future data analytical capabilities in the areas of neonatal decompensation, anemia of prematurity, apnea of prematurity, pain management, jaundice treatment, and retinopathy of prematurity. McMaster Children's Hospital in Montreal, Canada, Women and Infants' Hospital in Rhode Island, and international sites in China have also participated in the project team.

Fig. 4 diagrams the project's dynamic workflow, allowing data like that listed in **Table 5** to be collected and forwarded to online real-time analysis. Upon analysis, it is either presented back to the bedside through the user interface for clinical decision making or stored in its original format as well as newly generated analytics. This latter pathway is referred to as data persistency. The data mining phase allows examining of the larger and ever-growing database to generate new information specifically intended to support disease-specific research. Finally, the redeployment component yields new, clinically validated algorithms back to online analysis so that new incoming real-time data can continuously be compared and enhanced to yield earlier data informed predictions.[45]

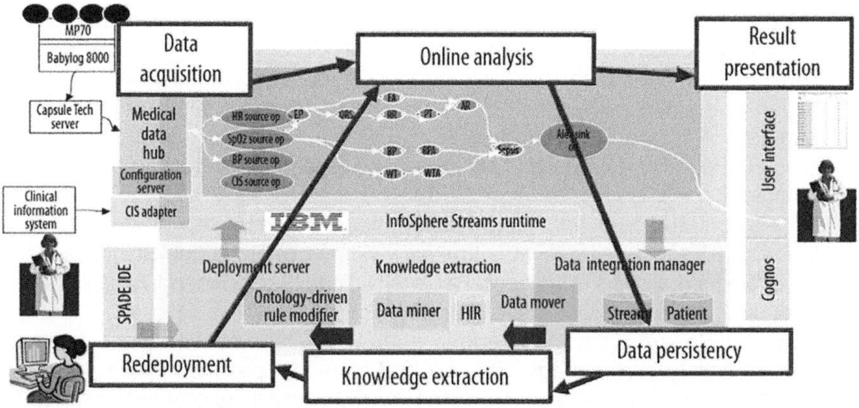

Fig. 4. Schematic of the Artemis Project. BP, blood pressure; CIS, clinical information system; HR, heart rate; SpO2, pulse oximetry.

SUMMARY

Although all of this holds great promise, the Artemis Project and other ventures like it are still in the feasibility stages with no direct impact on bedside care as yet. Expert researchers tied to the projects are comparing clinician observations and current evidence-based guidelines to existing patient outcomes. NICUs provide critical care for preterm, born before 37 weeks, and ill newborns. The costs are not insignificant. As recently as 2011, average length of stay for hospitals reporting to the National Perinatal Information Center was 13.2 days across all gestations and diagnoses.[20] Another source reports that 30% to 35% of NICU admissions have a length of stay of fewer than 4 days, whereas the remaining 65% to 70% have an average length of stay of about 20 days.[47] NICU patients account for 0.15% of the US population but consume about 0.45% of total US health care costs. Furthermore, NICU care accounts for 75% of all dollars spent for newborn care.[18,47] The goal of big data health care analytics in neonatal care is what it is and can be for other disciplines: to understand patterns existing in real-time physiologic data and laboratory values or other clinical studies, that could lead to prevention, enhanced triage, early detection of instability with deployment of early warnings, and reduction of readmissions. Equally important is a focus on cost reductions of health care, particularly in the US economy. Current spending levels are not sustainable. Although use of big data health care analytics may not provide all solutions as we move forward in the discipline of neonatology, it is interesting to realize that possibilities are within reach. Most importantly, the tiniest of patients entrusted to collective caregiving may achieve the reward of safe, cost-effective, timely outcomes to the medical challenges that faced them with birth.

REFERENCES

1. Schneider EC, Sarnak DO, Squires D, et al. Mirror, mirror 2017: international comparison reflects flaws and opportunities for better U.S. health care. The Commonwealth Fund; 2017. Available at: http://www.commonwealthfund.org/publications/fund-reports/2017/jul/mirror-mirror-international-comparisons-2017. Accessed February 12, 2018.
2. Hartman M, Martin AB, Espinosa N, et al. National healthcare spending in 2016: spending and enrollment growth slow after initial coverage expansion. Health Aff 2018;37(1):150–60. Available at: https://www.healthaffairs.org/doi/pdf/10.1377/hlthaff.2017.1299. Accessed December 16, 2017.
3. Dieleman JL, Squires E, Bui AL, et al. Factors associated with increases in US healthcare spending. JAMA 2017;318(17):1668–78.
4. Powell L. Why are healthcare costs so high in the USA versus other countries? Available at: https://www.focusforhealth.org/healthcare-costs-high-usa-versus-countries/. Accessed December 6, 2017.
5. Peter G. Peterson foundation. Healthcare. Available at: https://www.pgpf.org/finding-solutions/healthcare. Accessed December 16, 2017.
6. Centers for Medicare and Medicaid Services. National health expenditures: NHE fact sheet. Available at: https://www.cms.gov/Research-Statistics-Data-and-Systems/Statistics-Trends-and-Reports/NationalHealthExpendData/NHE-Fact-Sheet.html. Accessed December 16, 2017.
7. Bates DW, Saria A, Ohno-Machado L, et al. Big data in health care: using analytics to identify and manage high-risk and high-cost patients. Health Aff 2014;33(7):1123–31. Available at: https://www.healthaffairs.org/doi/pdf/10.1377/hlthaff.2014.0041. Accessed on February 12, 2016.

8. Raghupathi W, Raghupathi V. Big data analytics in healthcare: promise and potential. Health Inf Sci Syst 2014;2:3. Available at: https://www.ncbi.nlm.nih.gov/pmc/articles/PMC4341817/?report=reader. Accessed December 6, 2017.
9. Hilbert M, Lopez P. The world's technological capacity to store, communicate, and compute information. Science 2011;332(6025):60–5.
10. Mashey JR. Big data and the next wave of InfraStress. Slides from invited lecture, April 25, 1998. Usenix. Available at: http://static.usenix.org/event/usenix99/invited_talks/mashey.pdf. Accessed November 6, 2017.
11. Lohr S. The origins of 'big data': an etymological detective story. The New York Times 2013. Available at: https://bits.blogs.nytimes.com/2013/02/01/the-origins-of-big-data-an-etymological-detective-story/. Accessed February 6, 2018.
12. Parikh RB, Kakad M, Bates DW. Integrating predictive analytics into high-value care: the dawn of precision delivery. JAMA 2016;315(7):651–2.
13. Kruse CS, Goswamy R, Raval Y, et al. Challenges and opportunities of big data in health care: a systematic review. JMIR Med Inform 2016;4(4):e38. Eysenbach G, ed.
14. Murdoch TB, Detsky AS. The inevitable application of big data to health care. JAMA 2013;309(13):1351–2.
15. Martin JA, Hamilton BE, Sutton PD, et al. Births: final data for 2016. National vital statistics reports, vol. 67, no 1. Hyattsville (MD): National Center for Health Statistics; 2018. Available at: https://www.cdc.gov/nchs/products/nvsr.htm. Accessed on February 16, 2018.
16. Martin JA, Hamilton BE, Osterman MJK. Births in the United States, 2016. NCHS data brief, no 287. Hyattsville (MD): National Center for Health Statistics; 2018. Available at: https://www.cdc.gov/nchs/products/databriefs/db287.htm. Accessed on January 23, 2018.
17. Harrison W, Goodman D. Epidemiological trends in neonatal intensive care, 2007-2012. JAMA Pediatr 2015;169(9):855–62.
18. Bui AL, Dieleman JL, Hamavid H, et al. Spending on children's personal health care in the United States, 1996-2013. JAMA Pediatr 2017;171(2):181–9.
19. Available at: https://www.healthsystemtracker.org/chart-collection/health-expenditures-vary-across-population/?_sf_s=How+Do+Health+Expenditures+Vary+Across+the+Population#item-start. Accessed February 4, 2018.
20. March of dimes and national perinatal information center. Special care nursery admissions, 2011. Available at: https://www.marchofdimes.org/peristats/pdfdocs/nicu_summary_final.pdf. Accessed December 16, 2017.
21. Shulman J, Braun D, Lee HC, et al. Association between neonatal intensive care unit admission rates and illness acuity. JAMA Pediatr 2018;172(1):17–23.
22. Johnson TJ, Patel AL, Jegier B, et al. The cost of morbidities in very low birth-weight infants. J Pediatr 2013;162(2):243–9.e1.
23. Neidig JR, Megel ME, Koehler KM. The critical path: an evaluation of the applicability of nursing case management in the NICU. Neonatal Netw 1992;11(5):45–52.
24. Forsyth TJ, Maney LA, Ramirez A, et al. Nursing case management in the NICU. Neonatal Netw 1998;17(7):23–34.
25. Diehl-Svrjcek BC, Richardson R. Decreasing NICU costs in the managed care arena: the positive impact of collaborative high-risk OB and NICU disease management programs. Lippincotts Case Manag 2005;10(3):159–66.
26. Apgar V. The newborn (Apgar) scoring system: reflections and advice. Pediatr Clin North Am 1966;13(3):645–50.
27. Finster M, Wood M. The Apgar score has survived the test of time. Anesthesiology 2005;102(4):855–7.

28. Saria S, Rajani AK, Gould J, et al. Integration of early physiologic responses predicts later illness severity in preterm infants. Sci Transl Med 2010;2(48):48ra65.
29. Kurinczuk JJ, White-Koenig M, Badawi N. Epidemiology of neonatal encephalopathy and hypoxic-ischemic encephalopathy. Early Hum Dev 2010;86(6):329–38.
30. Mello M, Chandra A, Gawande A, et al. National costs of the medical liability system. Health Aff 2010;29(9):1569–77. Available at: https://www.healthaffairs.org/doi/pdf/10.1377/hlthaff.2009.0807. Accessed February 25.2018.
31. Kaiser permanente early-onset sepsis calculator. Available at: https://neonatalsepsiscalculator.kaiserpermanente.org/InfectionProbabilityCalculator.aspx. Accessed February 6, 2018.
32. Escobar GJ, Puopolo KM, Wi S, et al. Stratification of risk of early-onset sepsis in newborns > 34 weeks' gestation. Pediatrics 2014;133:30–6, 2011;128:e1155-63.
33. Puopolo KM, Draper D, Wi S, et al. Estimating the probability of neonatal early-onset infection on the basis of maternal risk factors. Pediatrics 2011;128(5):e1155–63.
34. Kuzniewicz MW, Walsh EM, Li S, et al. Development and implementation of an early-onset sepsis calculator to guide antibiotic management in late preterm and term neonates. Jt Comm J Qual Patient Saf 2016;42(5):232–9.
35. Kuzniewicz MW, Puopolo KM, Fischer A, et al. A quantitative, risk-based approach to the management of neonatal early-onset sepsis. JAMA Pediatr 2017;171(4):365–71.
36. University Hospitals Cleveland Medical Center. Available at: http://www.uhhospitals.org/cleveland/patients-and-visitors/billing-insurance-and-medical-records/patient-pricing-information. Accessed February 4, 2018.
37. Merriam webster online dictionary. Available at: https://www.merriam-webster.com/dictionary/decompensation. Accessed January 18, 2018.
38. Bohanon FJ, Mrazek AA, Shabana MT, et al. Heart rate variability analysis is more sensitive at identifying neonatal sepsis than conventional vital signs. Am J Surg 2015;210(4):661–7.
39. Fairchild KD. Predictive monitoring for early detection of sepsis in neonatal ICU patients. Curr Opin Pediatr 2013;25(2):172–9.
40. McIntosh N, Becher JC, Cunningham S, et al. Clinical diagnosis of pneumothorax is late: use of trend data and decision support might allow preclinical detection. Pediatr Res 2000;48(3):408–15.
41. Fabres J, Carlo WA, Phillips V, et al. Both extremes of arterial carbon dioxide pressure and the magnitude of fluctuations in arterial carbon dioxide pressure are associated with severe intraventricular hemorrhage in preterm infants. Pediatrics 2007;123(3):299–305.
42. Tuzcu V, Nas S, Ulusar U, et al. Altered heart rhythm dynamics in very low birth weight infants with impending intraventricular hemorrhage. Pediatrics 2009;123(3):810–5.
43. Shankaran S, Langer JS, Nadya Kazzi S, et al. Cumulative index of exposure to hypocarbia and hyperoxia as risk factors for periventricular leukomalacia in low birth weight infants. Pediatrics 2006;118(4):1654–9.
44. Society of Critical Care Medicine. Critical care statistics, 2018. Available at: http://www.sccm.org/Communications/Pages/CriticalCareStats.aspx. Accessed February 4, 2018.
45. McGregor C. Big data in the neonatal intensive care unit. Computer 2013;46(6):54–9.

46. Khazaei H, Mench-Bressan N, McGregor C, et al. Health informatics for neonatal intensive care units: an analytical modeling perspective. IEEE J Transl Eng Health Med 2015;3:1–9.
47. Kornhauser M, Schneiderman R. How plans can improve outcome and cut costs for preterm infant care. Manag Care 2010;19(1):28–30.

Fetal Surgery and Delayed Cord Clamping

Neonatal Implications

Karen M. Frank, DNP, RNC-NIC, APRN-CNS

KEYWORDS

- Delayed umbilical cord clamping • Premature newborn • Umbilical cord
- Fetal surgery • Fetoscopy

KEY POINTS

- Delayed umbilical cord clamping in the premature newborn provides an autologous transfusion of blood that helps with the transition to extrauterine life.
- Delayed umbilical cord clamping has a positive impact on morbidity, including anemia, hemodynamic instability, intraventricular hemorrhage, and necrotizing enterocolitis.
- Fetal therapy has an effect on morbidity and mortality for fetuses diagnosed with certain congenital anomalies.

INTRODUCTION

Advances in the last several decades in the care of the fetus have had a significant impact on the morbidity and mortality for these special patients. Delayed umbilical cord clamping (DCC) and fetal surgery have played a part in preventing morbidity and mortality as well as improving the quality of life for these infants.

DCC is recommended for both vigorous term and preterm newborns for at least 30 to 60 seconds by the American Academy of Pediatrics, the International Liaison Committee on Resuscitation, the International Consensus on Cardiopulmonary Resuscitation, and the American College of Obstetricians and Gynecologists.[1–6] The World Health Organization supports DCC as well, with the recommendation of waiting at least a full minute to assist in the prevention of iron deficiency anemia, especially in third-world countries.[7]

Fetal surgery or fetoscopy has become a viable option for fetuses with certain congenital defects. As a result of advances made in fetal ultrasound diagnosis and technology, fetal surgeries for the treatment of congenital diaphragmatic hernia (CDH), myelomeningocele, twin-to-twin transfusion syndrome, fetal lower urinary tract obstructions, amniotic band syndrome, and congenital cystic adenoid malformation or congenital pulmonary airway malformations has improved the quality of life and

---

Disclosure Statement: The author has nothing to disclose.
Department of Nursing, Towson University, LI 322, 8000 York Road, Towson, MD 21252, USA
E-mail address: kmfrank@towson.edu

Crit Care Nurs Clin N Am 30 (2018) 499–507
https://doi.org/10.1016/j.cnc.2018.07.006 ccnursing.theclinics.com

survival for these patients.[8] Although some of these therapies or surgeries remain a part of clinical trials and are not currently the standard of care they continue to show promise in the care of these patients.

BACKGROUND AND HISTORY

Delayed Umbilical Cord Clamping

Transition from fetal to newborn life is a normal physiologic process that has occurred since the beginning of time. Clamping the umbilical cord after birth is an intervention that must take place and assists the newborn in this transition. The timing of when to clamp the umbilical cord has varied throughout the centuries. "Primitive cultures" waited several hours to clamp the umbilical cord after delivery. Although not exactly known when this practice changed, based on available evidence it is believed that clamping the umbilical cord immediately after birth was being practiced in the early 17th century.[9]

In the last century, with advances in technology and the care of smaller, sicker newborns, immediate cord clamping (ICC), which consists of clamping the umbilical cord within the first 20 to 30 seconds after birth, has become a common practice in the United States. This practice has found to potentially deprive the newborn of an additional 7 to 10 mL/kg of blood volume, which can help in this transition.[10] However, a brief, 30- to 120-second delay in clamping the umbilical cord has been found to result in a placental transfusion that supplies the newborn with additional blood volume and iron-rich red blood cells.[11]

In a Cochrane review of full-term newborns who have received DCC compared with newborns who received ICC, there were no statistically significant differences in mortality rate, Apgar score, or admission to a neonatal intensive care unit.[12] There were many reported advantages to DCC including higher birth weight, increased hemoglobin values, and increased iron stores lasting up to 6 months after birth. DCC assists in the transition to extrauterine life that helps neonates of all gestational ages, but may be lifesaving to the vulnerable preterm neonate. DCC at birth can support the preterm newborn during the transition to extrauterine life through an autologous transfusion of blood from the placenta to the newborn. This intervention has been found to result in fewer transfusions for anemia, a decreased incidence of intraventricular hemorrhage (IVH), and a decreased incidence of necrotizing enterocolitis (NEC).[13] This article focuses on DCC in the premature newborn delivered at less than 37 weeks of gestation.

Fetal Surgery

Making an accurate fetal diagnosis is of the utmost importance with fetal surgery. Fetal surgeries began to be performed in the late 20th century as a result of improved fetal ultrasound techniques and the role they played in the accurate diagnosis of congenital anomalies that may benefit from fetal surgery.[14] Open fetal surgeries began in the 1960s to treat Rh isoimmunization when it was suspected that without the surgery the fetus would not survive. Although open fetal surgeries placed the mother at risk for morbidity, without intervention the fetus was expected to die during the birthing process or immediately afterward.[14] With advances in technology, percutaneous approaches replaced open procedures as a result of the better outcomes found with this technique.[14]

Fetal transfusions for the treatment of erythroblastosis fetalis for fetuses with Rh incompatibility were among the first fetal surgeries performed. Liley, the physician who introduced the technique, was able to determine fetal demise based on the spectrophotometric results from amniotic fluid samples obtained during amniocentesis.[14] In 1989, the first fetal surgery for diaphragmatic hernia was performed at the University of California, San Francisco.[15] Further studies explored different surgical techniques including tracheal occlusion and, although it allowed for expansion of the lung, it also reduced the number of type II cells and possibly inhibited surfactant production. Later techniques included the placement of a balloon that obstructed the trachea and allowed for lung growth, which became known as fetal endoscopic tracheal occlusion procedure. This procedure showed an increase in survival rates.[14]

There were several different types of surgical techniques performed, including open surgery, intraperitoneal, and intravascular transfusion.[14] Comparisons of the different techniques focused on the less invasive percutaneous techniques with the open surgical procedures, or more invasive techniques focusing mostly at the effects on the mother.[14] As percutaneous fetal transfusion therapies advanced and showed positive outcomes for the fetus, as well as limited risks to both the mother and the fetus, open surgical techniques were no longer practiced.[14]

Fetal surgery or fetoscopy has become a viable option for fetuses with congenital defects owing to advances in technology, including smaller optical systems for visualization, gas amniodistention, newer trocars, robotic systems, and advances in fetal ultrasound examinations.[8] Currently, there are fetal therapies for several congenital anomalies including myelomeningocele, twin-to-twin transfusion syndrome, fetal lower urinary tract obstructions, amniotic band syndrome, and congenital cystic adenoid malformation or congenital pulmonary airway malformations. The main complication of fetal surgery is preterm labor as a result of stimulation of the uterus during the surgical intervention. With the advancement of tocolytics and advances in minimally invasive fetoscopy techniques, the incidence of premature labor can be decreased. Many therapies are being performed at specialized centers and in ongoing research trials.

DELAYED UMBILICAL CORD CLAMPING FOR THE PREMATURE NEWBORN

Clinical Benefits

DCC has been shown to result in a 7 to 10 mL/kg autologous transfusion of blood for the premature newborn and has an impact on morbidity including anemia, hemodynamic instability, IVH, and NEC. Anemia affects growth, slows recovery, and places the neonate at risk of requiring blood transfusions. A systematic review and meta-analysis by Rabe and associates in 2008 examined waiting 30 to 120 seconds after birth to clamp the umbilical cord. The DCC group had higher hematocrit values after birth (5 studies; $P = .0007$), a decreased number of newborns required transfusions (3 studies; $P = .005$), and, when they did require transfusions, they needed a lesser number of transfusions (4 studies; $P = .0004$).[16] Similar results were found by other investigators as well, including higher hematocrit values with a 30- to 120-second delay in cord clamping.[17–20]

Hypotension is another issue commonly seen in the premature neonate, which can be a result of not receiving the autologous transfusion of blood from the placenta to the newborn. Hemodynamic instability is thought to cause the hypotension and occurs in more than one-half of premature neonates. This hemodynamic instability is thought to be linked to the incidence of IVH.[21,22]

The structure called the germinal matrix in the premature neonate is the anatomic site where neural cells develop. This highly vascular and metabolically active structure can be damaged easily, resulting in IVH. The premature neonate also has a pressure-passive cerebral circulation with an impaired ability to autoregulate cerebral brain blood flow. This inability to autoregulate can cause fluctuations in the systemic blood pressure leading to the occurrence of IVH. In a study by Rabe and colleagues,[16,23] the investigators found a decrease in the incidence of IVH (7 studies; $P = .002$) in premature neonates who received DCC compared with the neonates who received ICC. Similar results were found in a randomized, controlled trial by Elimian and colleagues[18] in neonates delivered between 24 to 34 weeks of gestation. The study showed that the premature newborns who received DCC had higher initial hemoglobin (17.4 ± 2.5 g/dL vs 16.3 ± 2.3 g/dL; $P = .001$) and hematocrit values (51.3 ± 7.3 vs 47.4 ± 7.3; $P = .001$) compared with the premature newborns who received ICC.

There is an association between infants who receive blood transfusions for anemia and the incidence of NEC, the most common gastrointestinal emergency seen in the premature neonate. A Cochrane review found that premature newborns who received DCC compared with those who received ICC had a decrease in the incidence of NEC (5 trials including 241 infants; relative risk, 0.62; 95% confidence interval, 0.43–0.90).[23] Aziz and colleagues[19] (2012) found similar results when performing DCC for 45 seconds (1.3% vs 5.4%; $P = .026$; n = 480).

Perceived Risks

Concerns have been brought to the forefront regarding DCC on the premature newborn because it may cause a delay in resuscitation and an increased need for treatment for hyperbilirubinemia. Aziz and colleagues[19] studied newborns delivered at less than 33 weeks of gestation and reported no differences in mortality, Apgar score, and delivery room ventilation in premature newborns who received DCC compared with ICC. This finding supports the idea that the performance of DCC does not have a negative impact on resuscitation of the premature newborn and the benefits of DCC do outweigh the potential risks.

As a result of the increased duration of transfer time of the premature newborn to the radiant warmer from the time of delivery when DCC is performed, it was thought that thermoregulation may be negatively affected causing hypothermia. Rabe and coworkers found no differences in admission temperatures in the premature newborns who received DCC compared with those who received ICC. It is important to note the DCC time varied in length from 30 seconds to a maximum time of 120 seconds.[13] Aziz and colleagues[19] performed DCC for 45 seconds and reported no differences in admission temperatures between premature newborns who received DCC and ICC. Interestingly, DCC may also result in an increase in the newborn's body temperature per a study by Jelin and colleagues.[24] In this study, Jelin and colleagues found that performing DCC for 30 to 60 seconds resulted in an increase in body temperature in the newborns who received DCC from 36.3°C (before DCC) to 36.5°C (after DCC).

Hyperbilirubinemia is another concern related to the autologous transfusion of blood by the placenta to the newborn during DCC. A Cochrane review found higher peak bilirubin concentrations in newborns who received a longer placental transfusion compared with a shorter transfusion time (7 trials that included 320 infants; Mean Deviation, 15.01 mmol/L; 95% confidence interval, 5.62–24.40). There was a trend toward a need for treatment with phototherapy as reported by 3 studies (180 infants; relative risk, 1.21; 95% confidence interval, 0.94–1.55), although it did not reach statistical significance.[23]

Duration of Time Between Birth and Clamping the Umbilical Cord

The optimal duration of time from when the premature newborn is delivered to clamping the umbilical cord remains undecided, with the time ranging from 30 to 180 seconds, as indicated by 2 Cochrane reviews.[13,16] However, the American Academy of

Pediatrics currently supports the American College of Obstetricians and Gynecologists in the recommendation of waiting at least 30 to 60 seconds after birth before clamping the umbilical cord for both vigorous term and preterm newborns[1,2]; the World Health Organization recommends waiting at least 60 seconds after birth before clamping the umbilical cord.[7]

Exclusion Criteria

There are circumstances where DCC may be contraindicated as a result of a maternal condition or the need to resuscitate the newborn immediately after birth. Some studies excluded multiple gestation deliveries,[19,22,25] whereas other studies such as the one by Kugelman and colleagues[26] included multiples in their studies and found no complications. Several of the studies excluded neonates with congenital malformations, severe intrauterine growth retardation, cord prolapse, discordant twins, and maternal conditions such as bleeding and maternal substance abuse.[19,22,26]

TYPES OF FETAL SURGERY

Twin-to-Twin Transfusion Syndrome

Twin-to-twin transfusion syndrome can occur when twins share the same placenta and there is an unbalanced flow of blood that results in one twin becoming the donor and the other twin being the recipient. Twin-to-twin transfusion syndrome occurs in approximately 15% of all monochorionic pregnancies. It can be identified on fetal ultrasound examination by polyhydramnios in one sac and oligohydramnios in the other sac.[27] Twin-to-twin transfusion syndrome diagnosed before 26 weeks of gestation has a high morbidity and mortality rate and if left untreated mortality rates may be as high as 95%.[28] Laser photocoagulation therapy has shown to be the best treatment for twin-to-twin transfusion syndrome and is recommended as the first line of treatment. In a study by the Senat group, there was a decrease in cystic periventricular leukomalacia and a decreased incidence of neurologic complications at 6 months of age in the fetuses who received fetal therapy.[29] There are diagnostic criteria used to determine which fetuses would benefit from fetoscopic laser coagulation therapy. These criteria include no associated morphologic alterations, a normal karyotype, and no cervical modifications.[29] Fetoscopic laser coagulation surgery after 26 weeks gestational age is controversial related to pulmonary maturation, amniodrainage, and premature delivery compared with newborns who have had laser therapy, which showed a decrease in morbidity.[30] Premature rupture of the membranes is the main complication of fetoscopic laser coagulation therapy, with detachment of the placenta and chorioamnionitis being less common.[30]

Congenital Diaphragmatic Hernia

CDH occurs in the fetus when there is an opening in the diaphragm, allowing parts of the bowel, stomach, and liver to move into the chest cavity. When CDH occurs, it compresses the lungs of the fetus, affecting the ability of the lungs to develop normally causing hypoplasia. Survival of CDH is based on the amount of lung hypoplasia, which can be determined by the lung–head ratio or fetal MRI volumetry. Fetoscopic endotracheal occlusion therapy is a technique where a balloon is placed endoscopically in the trachea under local anesthesia temporarily to expand the lungs and prevent further damage.[14] This procedure can be observed in this video: https://www.hopkinsmedicine.org/gynecology_obstetrics/specialty_areas/fetal_therapy/fetal_interventions_procedures/fetoscopic_tracheal_occlusion.html.

Fetal ex utero intrapartum treatment procedures were initially performed at delivery to remove the balloon; however, fetoscopic removal of the tracheal balloon proved more successful with a 65% survival rate compared with 8% if left untreated.[31] Peiró and colleagues[8] stated that the average surgical time to perform the therapy was 26 minutes. The procedure was performed on fetuses with gestational ages between 26 and 28 weeks who displayed severe pulmonary hypoplasia, a lung–head ratio of less than 1, and herniation of the liver into the chest cavity, as indicated on prenatal ultrasound examination. Two weeks after the tracheal occlusion, there was a noted increase in the lung–head ratio value as well as fetal lung volume. Premature rupture of the membranes, however, occurred in 30% of the cases. Failure of the human amnion to heal may result in ongoing amniotic fluid leakage after fetal intervention, resulting in premature delivery and increased morbidity and mortality. Fetal surgery for CDH remains controversial and is performed only at specialized centers in the United States.[8]

Fetal Lower Urinary Tract Obstruction

Fetal lower urinary tract obstruction or obstructive uropathy often leads to oligohydramnios which causes pulmonary hypoplasia. The most common cause is posturethral valves seen in male fetuses. The degree of obstructive uropathy varies significantly in severity. The most severe causes are associated with decreased amniotic fluid, which leads to pulmonary hypoplasia and may cause death in the newborn.[8] If there is normal renal function in the fetus, decompression of the bladder can preserve renal function and decrease morbidity and mortality. It is important to determine renal function by taking serial fetal urine samples from the kidneys, bladder, and ureters. If renal function in the fetus with obstructive uropathy is satisfactory, the percutaneous placement of a pigtail catheter, a vesicoamniotic shunt, or vesicostomy by fetoscopic or open fetal surgery can be performed.[32] Newer, minimally invasive therapy includes fetal cystoscopy where the ablation of the valves is performed using a YAG laser that passes through the cystoscope and dilates the posterior urethra. Concerns with this therapy include kidney and bladder function. Postnatal survival is approximately 40% to 50% for normal renal function using the vesicoamniotic shunting technique and 65% to 75% for the fetal cystoscopy.[33]

Amniotic Band Syndrome

Amniotic band syndrome causes constriction of a fetal extremity, which can lead to loss of function or constriction of the umbilical cord, which can lead to death. The severity of amniotic band syndrome can be mild, such as seen in pseudosyndactyly, a mitten-type deformity of hands and feet. It can also be severe, resulting in limb amputation or defects in the body wall. Fetal ultrasound examination can be used to detect limb involvement. The affected limb will show edema distally. Treatment involves fetoscopic lysis of the band, which can preserve a limb; if the umbilical cord is affected, it can prevent death.[8]

Sacrococcygeal Teratoma

Sacrococcygeal teratoma develops in utero in the sacrococcygeal region located at the base of the spine. Sacrococcygeal teratoma is diagnosed by fetal ultrasound examination and has a high risk of perinatal morbidity and mortality. Most tumors are benign, but can grow quite large. The larger the teratoma the greater risk for high-output cardiac failure and fetal or neonatal death. Fetal surgery may be offered if the fetus is still previable and has developed hydrops and or cardiac insufficiency.[8] A study by Van Mieghem and colleagues[34] showed that fetal therapy improved perinatal outcomes for fetuses with a solid tumor who developed hydrops. Complications associated with the fetal therapy included fetal death and premature birth. Although Hecher and Hackeloer performed successful fetoscopic treatment using a laser on a narrow-based teratoma,[35] other authors reported necrosis of the vagina, anus, and bladder owing to the close proximity of the teratoma and the genitals in their studies.[36] Surgical removal after birth is necessary for these tumors.

Myelomeningocele

Neural tube defects are a result of a midline vertebral defect occurring most frequently in the lumbosacral vertebrae during fetal development. A myelomeningocele can have a large impact on quality of life, leading to neurologic dysfunction, urinary and fecal incontinence, skeletal deformities, and sexual dysfunction later in life. A fetus with myelomeningocele has a 90% chance of developing hydrocephalus. Decompression of the brain in the fetus who has developed hydrocephalus may preserve function and can have a major impact on outcome. It is also thought that continued trauma in utero to the exposed spinal cord can lead to neurologic impairment. Covering the exposed cord in utero can help to prevent this damage. Myelomeningocele can be diagnosed early in gestation through fetal ultrasound examination. Research shows the earlier the intervention, the less the morbidity.[37] Current fetal therapy includes covering the defect with a patch. An ongoing trial, Management of Myelomeningocele (MOM), compares infants who have received treatment in utero with infants who received treatment after delivery.

SUMMARY

Delayed Umbilical Cord Clamping in the Premature Newborn

DCC is recommended for both vigorous term and preterm newborns for at least 30 to 60 seconds by the American Academy of Pediatrics, the International Liaison Committee on Resuscitation, the International Consensus on Cardiopulmonary Resuscitation, and the American College of Obstetricians and Gynecologists[1–5] and for at least 60 seconds by the World Health Organization.[7] The benefits of DCC include increased hemoglobin values, increased iron stores lasting up to 6 months after birth, and a decreased incidence of IVH and NEC; it has no impact on mortality rate, Apgar score, or admission to a neonatal intensive care unit. The benefits far outweigh the risks. The only potential complication associated with DCC is hyperbilirubinemia, which may require phototherapy.

Fetal Surgery

Fetal therapies have shown success in the treatment of twin-to-twin transfusion syndrome, amniotic band syndrome, severe CDH, and posterior urethral valves. Progress continues to be made on other types of congenital anomalies. Premature rupture of the membranes and preterm delivery remain potential complications of fetoscopic treatment. However, with technologic advances, improvements in practitioner skill levels, and collaboration between obstetricians and pediatric surgeons, there is promise for improved outcomes related to these anomalies.

REFERENCES

1. Committee of Obstetric Practice. Delayed umbilical cord clamping after birth. Committee Opinion. 2017. Available at: https://www.acog.org/-/media/Committee-Opinions/Committee-on-Obstetric-Practice/co684.pdf?dmc=1&ts=20180105T1520246390. Accessed January 3, 2018.
2. American Academy of Pediatrics. Delayed umbilical cord clamping after birth. Pediatrics 2017;139(6). https://doi.org/10.1542/peds.2017-0957.
3. Committee of Obstetric Practice. Timing of umbilical cord clamping after birth. Obstet Gynecol 2012;120(6):1522–6.

4. International Liaison Committee on Resuscitation. The international liaison committee on resuscitation (ILCOR) consensus on science with treatment recommendations for pediatric and neonatal patients: neonatal resuscitation. Pediatrics 2006;117(5):E978–88.
5. Perlman J, Wyllie J, Kattwinkel J, et al. 2010 International consensus on cardiopulmonary resuscitation and emergency cardiovascular care science with treatment recommendations. Circulation 2010;122(suppl 2):S516–38.
6. Raju T. Don't rush to cut the cord: new recommendations call for delayed cord clamping in preterm infants. AAP News 2013;34(4):17.
7. World Health Organization. Optimal time of cord clamping for the prevention of iron deficiency anemia in infants. 2017. Available at: http://www.who.int/elena/titles/cord_clamping/en/. Accessed January 3, 2018.
8. Peiró J, Carreras E, Guillén G, et al. Therapeutic indications of fetoscopy: a five year institutional experience. J Laparoendosc Adv Surg Tech A 2009;19(2):229–37.
9. Inch S. Management of the third stage of labour-another cascade of intervention? Midwifery 1984;1:114–22.
10. Ghavam S, Batra D, Mercer J, et al. Effects of placental transfusion in extremely low birth weight infants: meta-analysis of long- and short-term outcomes. Transfusion 2014. https://doi.org/10.1111/trf.12469.
11. Hutton E, Hassan E. Late vs early clamping of the umbilical cord in full-term neonates. JAMA 2007;297(11):1241–52.
12. McDonald SJ, Middleton P, Dowswell T, et al. Effect of timing of umbilical cord clamping of term infants on maternal and neonatal outcomes. Cochrane Database Syst Rev 2013;7:1–195.
13. Rabe H, Reynolds G, Diaz-Rossello J. Early versus delayed umbilical cord clamping in preterm infants. The Cochrane Collaboration 2010;2:1–32.
14. Kitagawa H, Pringle KC. Fetal surgery: a critical review. Pediatr Surg Int 2017;33:421–33.
15. Harrison MR, Langer JC, Adzick NS, et al. Correction of congenital diaphragmatic hernia *in utero*, v. initial clinical experience. J Pediatr Surg 1990;25:47–55.
16. Rabe H, Reynolds G, Diaz-Rossello J. A systematic review and meta-analysis of a brief delay in clamping the umbilical cord of preterm infants. Neonatology 2008;93:138–44.
17. Baenziger O, Stolkin F, Keel M, et al. The influence of the timing of cord clamping on postnatal cerebral oxygenation in preterm neonates: a randomized controlled trial. Pediatrics 2006;119:455–9.
18. Elimian A, Goodman J, Escobedo M, et al. A randomized controlled trial of immediate versus delayed cord clamping in the preterm neonate. Am J Obstet Gynecol 2013;208(1):S22.
19. Aziz K, Chinnery H, Lacaze-Masmonteil T. A single-center experience of implementing delayed cord clamping in babies born at less than 33 weeks' gestational age. Adv Neonatal Care 2012;12(6):371–6.
20. Oh W, Fanaroff A, Carol W, et al, for the entire Eunice Kennedy Shriver National Institute of Child Health and Human Development Neonatal Research Network. Effects of delayed cord clamping in the very-low-birth-weight infants. J Perinatol 2011;31:S68–71.
21. Noori S, Stavroudis T, Seri I. Systemic and cerebral hemodynamics during the transitional period after premature birth. Clin Perinatol 2009;21:723–36.
22. Sommers R. Hemodynamic effects of delayed cord clamping in premature infants. Pediatrics 2012;129(3):E667–72.

23. Rabe H, Diaz-Rosello J, Duley L, et al. Effect of timing of umbilical cord clamping and other strategies to influence placental transfusion at preterm birth on maternal and infant outcomes. Cochrane Database Syst Rev 2012;8:84.
24. Jelin A, Zlatnik M, Kuppermann M, et al. Does a delayed cord clamping policy improve neonatal outcomes? Am J Obstet Gynecol 2014;210(1):S406.
25. Kaempf J, Tomlinson M, Kaempf A, et al. Delayed umbilical cord clamping in premature neonates. Obstet Gynecol 2012;120(2):325–30.
26. Kugelman A, Borenstein-Levin L, Riskin A, et al. Immediate versus delayed umbilical cord clamping in premature neonates born <35 weeks: a prospective, randomized, controlled trial. Am J Perinatol 2007;24:307–16.
27. Chasen ST, Al-Kouaty HB, Ballabh P, et al. Outcomes of dichorionic triplet pregnancies. Am J Obstet Gynecol 2002;186:765–7.
28. De Lia JE. Surgery of the placenta and umbilical cord. Clin Obstet Gynecol 1996; 39:607–25.
29. Senat MV, Deprest J, Boulvain M, et al. Endoscopic laser surgery versus serial amnioreduction for severe twin-to-twin transfusion syndrome. N Engl J Med 2004;351:136–44.
30. Middeldorp JM, Lopiore E, Sueters M, et al. Twin-to-twin transfusion syndrome after 26 weeks of gestation: is there a role for fetoscopic surgery? BJOG 2007; 114:694–8.
31. Jani J, Gratacós E, Greenough A, et al, and the FETO Task Group. Percutaneous fetal endoscopic tracheal occlusion (FETO) for severe left-sided congenital diaphragmatic hernia. Clin Obstet Gynecol 2005;48:910–22.
32. Tsao K, Albanese CT. Prenatal surgery for obstructive uropathy. World J Surg 2003;27:62–7.
33. Holmes N, Harrison MR, Baskin LS. Fetal surgery for posterior urethral valves: long-term postnatal outcomes. Pediatrics 2001;108:7.
34. Van Mieghem T, Al-Ibrahim A, Deprest J, et al. Minimally invasive therapy for fetal sacroccygeal teratoma: case series and systematic review. Ultrasound Obstet Gynecol 2014;43(6):611–9.
35. Hecher K, Hackeloer BJ. Intrauterine endoscopic laser surgery for fetal Sacrococcygeal teratoma. Lancet 1996;347(8999):470.
36. Graf JL, Albanese CT, Jennings RW, et al. Successful fetal sacrococcygeal teratoma resection in a hydroptic fetus. J Pediatr Surg 2000;35:1489–91.
37. Meuli M, Meuli-Simmen C, Hutchins G, et al. In utero surgery rescues neurological function at birth in sheep with spina bifida. Nat Med 1995;1:342–7.

[illegible]

Neonatal Encephalopathy

Current Management and Future Trends

Elizabeth A. Schump, MSN, ARNP, NNP-BC

KEYWORDS

• Neonatal • Newborn • Hypoxic ischemic encephalopathy • Therapeutic hypothermia

KEY POINTS

- If therapeutic hypothermia is begun before 6 hours of age, the progression of hypoxic ischemic encephalopathy is slowed.
- Infants suffering from hypoxic ischemic encephalopathy are at an increased risk for neurologic developmental delays and death, but have better outcomes if treated with therapeutic hypothermia.
- Management during therapeutic hypothermia should include amplitude-integrated electroencephalography, MRI, and near-infrared spectroscopy if available to help determine long-term outcomes.
- Many therapies are being researched that could enhance therapeutic hypothermia.

Hypoxic ischemic encephalopathy (HIE) can have lifelong consequences for infants suffering from it and their families. Most recent literature estimates neonatal deaths from HIE account for 23% of all neonatal deaths worldwide.[1] Based on the average of 4,000,000 births per year in the United States, as many as 12,000 infants are affected by HIE annually nationwide.[2] It is globally accepted that infants with HIE benefit from therapeutic hypothermia (TH), but the delivery method can vary widely. In this review, qualification criteria for TH, different treatment strategies, and future ideas for neuroprotection are covered.

PATHOPHYSIOLOGY OF HYPOXIC ISCHEMIC ENCEPHALOPATHY AND THERAPEUTIC HYPOTHERMIA

HIE is defined as acute or subacute perinatal asphyxia as evidenced by neurologic examination and laboratory data. It stems from decreased fetal cerebral blood flow (CBF) and/or hypoxemia.[1] Many perinatal events are associated with significantly reduced fetal CBF, the most common being placental abruption, umbilical cord prolapse or

Disclosure: The author has nothing to disclose.
Overland Park Regional Medical Center, NICU, 10500 Quivira Road, Overland Park, KS 66215, USA
E-mail address: bethgrady@hotmail.com

Crit Care Nurs Clin N Am 30 (2018) 509–521
https://doi.org/10.1016/j.cnc.2018.07.007 ccnursing.theclinics.com

true knot, uterine rupture, vasa previa, and nuchal cord. Occasionally, the cause of asphyxia is unknown, but if signs of HIE are present, TH should be initiated.

The natural progression of HIE occurs over several hours to days. The initial ischemic event causes a varying degree of immediate neuronal cell death owing to rapid depletion of high-energy metabolites, leading to depolarization of cells and cellular edema. Concurrently, the infant experiences a compensatory phase in which cardiac output is redirected to protect vital organs including the brain, myocardium, and adrenals. CBF and blood pressure are initially increased owing to epinephrine release. Unfortunately, these compensatory mechanisms quickly fail, leading to diminished cardiac output and CBF. Cerebral vascular autoregulation is lost, and CBF becomes dependent on systemic blood pressure, resulting in initial energy failure and further brain injury. Approximately 1 hour after this initial insult, a latent phase begins. Partial recovery of cerebral oxidative metabolism occurs. Cerebral autoregulation is restored and reperfusion begins. The neonate experiences a transient recovery period and may seem to improve. This latent phase continues for 6 to 15 hours before progressing to a secondary energy failure state. This final stage is often characterized by seizures, brain edema, and cellular apoptosis, and becomes increasingly severe for the first 24 to 48 hours. It can persist for several days before starting to improve.[3,4]

TH disrupts this cascade of events if started before secondary energy failure. Because this usually occurs at 6 to 15 hours of age, TH should be initiated as early as possible, but at least before 6 hours of age. If begun early, TH works in many ways to decrease the consequences of HIE. It reduces cellular metabolic demands and the accumulation of oxygen free radicals in addition to decreasing inflammation caused by brain injury.[3,4]

QUALIFICATION CRITERIA FOR THERAPEUTIC HYPOTHERMIA

Criteria have been established to identify infants who would benefit from TH[5–7] (Appendix 1). When these criteria are met, infants should be evaluated for encephalopathy. The Modified Sarnat Staging for HIE is commonly used for determining the degree of encephalopathy. With this tool, encephalopathy is delineated into mild, moderate, and severe categories.[8] It differs from the original Sarnat Staging because it does not include electroencephalogram (EEG) findings as part of the diagnostic criteria. With a great number of babies born at outlying hospitals and requiring transport to a tertiary center for TH, EEG is not a feasible option for determining the degree of encephalopathy before transport owing to a lack of resources. Also, TH should not be delayed while waiting to obtain an EEG.

The Thompson Scoring Tool was introduced in 1997 and provides an alternative to the Modified Sarnat Scoring system. Despite their many similarities, an advantage of this tool is the use of numeric values to determine the severity of HIE. A score of greater than 7 is the entry criteria for TH (**Table 1**). In clinical trials, neonates with higher Thompson scores had more abnormal amplitude-integrated EEG (aEEG) background patterns. Also, a score of 11 or greater was predictive of an adverse outcome such as death, cerebral palsy (CP), severe hearing or visual impairments, or neurodevelopmental delays.[9] A separate study found that a Thompson score of 12 or greater was associated with death before hospital discharge and/or severe epilepsy.[10]

MANAGEMENT DURING THERAPEUTIC HYPOTHERMIA

Although accepted for nearly a decade that TH improves outcomes for infants with HIE, debate over the best delivery method remains. Traditionally, neonates suffering from HIE who received whole body cooling at 33.5°C for 72 hours have a significantly

Table 1
Thompson scoring tool for hypoxic ischemic encephalopathy

	Score			
Sign	**0**	**1**	**2**	**3**
Tone	Normal	Increased	Decreased	Flaccid
Level of consciousness	Normal	Hyper alert	Lethargic	Comatose
Seizures	None	Minimal (<3/h)	>2/h	
Posture	Normal	Fisting/cycling	Strong distal flexion	Decerebrate
Moro reflex	Normal	Incomplete	Absent	
Grasp	Normal	Weak	Absent	
Suck	Normal	Weak	Absent with or without biting	
Respirations	Normal	Hyperventilation	Occasional apnea	Apnea
Fontanelle	Normal	Full, not tense	Tense	

Total Score: ________.
Mild encephalopathy: 1 to 10.
Moderate encephalopathy: 11 to 14.
Severe encephalopathy: 15 to 22.

reduced rate of death and disability.[11] However, in 1 study, cooling infants to 32°C and/or for up to 120 hours was evaluated for efficiency, but was prematurely closed owing to safety and futility concerns. This research showed that cooling for longer periods or at lower temperatures is not effective at decreasing the rate of death or disability, and may be more detrimental.[12]

A handful of studies have also been conducted that compare selective head cooling (SHC) versus whole body cooling. Most of these studies did not offer follow-up data, but ultimately produced the same results. No significant differences in morbidity or mortality were noted between the 2 groups.[13–16] On a larger scale, 3 different types of TH have been examined, including SHC, body cooling, and head and body cooling, also known as whole body cooling. In general, most of these studies focused on TH versus standard intensive care and did not compare the different methods of TH. Ultimately, the findings in each study supported the beneficial effects of TH over standard intensive care regardless of the type of TH used. However, most of these trials chose to use whole body cooling, making this method the most widely studied technique.[4–6,11,17,18] Whole body cooling has a few advantages over SHC, including easier access for aEEG, EEG, and MRI, which are important aspects of the TH process. Regardless of the type of TH used, a strict protocol including evidence-based practices should be followed to ensure the best outcome.

NEUROLOGIC MANAGEMENT

TH is a process centered around care of the neonatal brain, so the neurologic management during the cooling process is extensive. It begins shortly after birth with a thorough neurologic examination as described previously. Neurologic assessments should be completed throughout the TH process at a minimum of every 12 hours, and should be recorded as mild, moderate, or severe. These assessments, coupled with aEEG tracings, MRI, and near-infrared spectroscopy (NIRS) can shed some light on expected outcomes.

Multiple studies have investigated the usefulness of aEEG in determining long-term outcomes for infants suffering from HIE treated with TH. An aEEG is a form of raw EEG tracing that displays time-compressed minimum and maximum peak-to-peak amplitude variability. In healthy, term newborns, the amplitude should fluctuate between 10 and 40 μV depending on the infant's sleep–wake cycling. This pattern is called continuous normal voltage. In contrast, neonates suffering from HIE can show abnormal patterns on aEEG including discontinuous normal voltage, burst suppression, continuous low voltage, or flat tracing (FT; **Table 2**). FT demonstrates minimal brain activity, which can cause electrodes to display cardiac activity instead. To the untrained eye, these spikes may resemble seizures, but on closer examination, they are actually electrocardiogram waves.[19,20]

Most studies that have assessed the predictive value of aEEG have classified continuous normal voltage and discontinuous normal voltage tracings as normal or mildly abnormal, and burst suppression, continuous low voltage, and FT as abnormal, with FT being the most severe.[19,20] When the aEEG is normal at 6 hours of age, the likelihood of adverse neurodevelopmental outcomes and/or death is low, but an abnormal aEEG at 6 hours is not necessarily predictive of poor outcomes. However, there is an association between an abnormal aEEG at 48 hours and adverse neurodevelopmental outcomes and death in infants treated with TH.[21–23]

Video EEG is another form of EEG monitoring. Video EEG combines an EEG with real-time video recording of the infant. This method is useful in correlating clinical seizures with electrographic seizures, but is not commonly used in patients undergoing TH to date.

NIRS provides another type of cerebral monitoring that is, gaining attention owing to its noninvasive monitoring of cerebral tissue oxygenation, and its ease of use in conjunction with aEEG. Regional cerebral oxygenation and cerebral tissue oxygen extraction are continuously recorded while a NIRS monitor is in place. Regional cerebral oxygenation is a measure of oxygen supply to the brain, and cerebral tissue oxygen extraction shows the use of oxygen in the brain. In healthy, term newborns, there is a balance between the amount of oxygen supplied to the brain and the use of that oxygen, but this balance is often lost in infants with HIE.[24,25] Multiple studies have demonstrated that the combination of aEEG and NIRS has both a high positive and negative predictive value of determining short- and long-term outcomes after HIE.[24,26,27]

HIE is the number one cause of seizures in neonates. Infants presenting with moderate or severe HIE often have associated seizures, although the incidence is lower in those treated with TH.[28] They are caused by excessive depolarization of neurons and a shift in cell energy.[29] Seizures on aEEG will appear as a sudden increase in the minimum and maximum amplitude resembling an arch, with repetitive spikes or sharp waves on raw EEG lasting longer than 10 seconds.[20,30] Some of these are also

Table 2
aEEG tracings

Pattern	Type	Min Amp (mV)	Max Amp (mV)
CNV	Normal	10	40
DNV	Mildly abnormal	<5	>10
BS	Abnormal	<5	>25
CLV	Abnormal	<5	<10
FT	Severely abnormal	<5	<5

Abbreviations: BS, burst suppression; CLV, continuous low voltage; CNV, continuous normal voltage; DNV, discontinuous normal voltage; FT, flat tracing.

accompanied by clinical seizures; likewise, there are times when clinical seizures are not expressed on aEEG owing to the limited number of channels. In a small study, the median age at which seizures began was 13.1 hours. The maximum seizure burden was seen at 19.4 hours and the seizures continued for about 16.5 hours. Infants diagnosed with severe HIE had a significantly higher seizure burden than those with moderate HIE. Phenobarbital is considered the first-line antiepileptic drug (AED). When seizures are first recognized, a loading dose is given, and is repeated with 1 to 2 boluses if the seizures continue. Often, neonatal seizures are resistant to mono-AED treatment and a second-line AED is needed. In this case, either phenytoin or midazolam is usually the drug of choice. The likelihood of requiring a second line AED is significantly higher in patients with severe HIE compared with those with moderate HIE.[30]

The pattern of brain injury in infants with HIE differs depending on the severity and duration of the event. Predominantly, gray matter structures are affected in term infants. In less severe, but prolonged asphyxia, the hippocampus and cerebral cortex are typically compromised. These structures are both responsible for memory formation, but the hippocampus also converts long-term memory into permanent memory and helps with spatial navigation. In more severe, acute events, the basal ganglia and thalamus are usually affected the most, but there can also be damage to the brainstem. The basal ganglia regulates the initiation of movements, balance, and posture. Damage to this area also affects cognitive and emotional behaviors and can be linked to addictive behaviors and habit formation. The thalamus is responsible for perception, attention, and movement, and is important for maintaining alertness. Injury to either or both of these areas can also lead to CP. In severe, prolonged, perinatal asphyxia, all gray matter structures are usually affected.[31]

MRI with magnetic resonance spectroscopy (MRS) is a useful tool in determining long-term outcomes for infants with HIE. MRI with MRS illustrates these structural changes, as well as biochemical and metabolic changes that occur in the brain as a result of HIE. The biggest controversy over MRI/MRS is the timing of the study. It was originally thought that MRI should be performed no earlier than 1 week of age when brain swelling had most likely decreased enough to show structural changes.[32] However, with advances in MRI/MRS technology, including the evolution of diffusion-weighted imaging (DWI) sequences, the trend is moving toward obtaining the study at 4 to 6 days of age.[33] DWI was introduced in 1985 and has continued to evolve as a useful tool in determining long-term outcomes. Diffusion occurs when molecules move in a system. When movement of these molecules is limited in any direction, restricted diffusion occurs, and the DWI will appear bright.[34] Restricted diffusion can be caused by a number of abnormalities, with ischemia being the most common cause in infants with HIE. To help quantify the amount of diffusion present in a DWI image, an apparent diffusion coefficient is calculated. In a large metaanalysis, apparent diffusion coefficient values had a high sensitivity and specificity (79% and 85% respectively) in predicting neurologic outcome.[35]

MRS is often done in conjunction with MRI to look at lactate and *N*-acetyl aspartate levels. Peaks in lactate reflect tissue ischemia, and low *N*-acetyl aspartate peaks are seen when there is neuronal injury. Although the specificity with MRS is low, it can be somewhat useful if used in conjunction with MRI to determine possible neurologic outcomes.[19]

Along with monitoring neurologic status, sedation is also an important part of the TH process because it decreases shivering and increases comfort levels for patients. Morphine and fentanyl are the most common drugs of choice for sedation during TH. With each, a loading dose is usually given, followed by a continuous infusion.

These drugs have a decreased clearance rate during TH, and can become toxic quickly if they are not decreased or discontinued shortly after rewarming or with any signs of toxicity.[36–38]

TEMPERATURE MANAGEMENT

There are a handful of different cooling devices that provide TH for neonates. Regardless of which system is used, the infant should be placed on the cooling blanket as quickly as possible after the decision to cool has been made. A rectal temperature is obtained initially, and then an esophageal or rectal probe is placed for the duration of treatment to monitor core temperature continuously. A radiograph should be obtained to confirm placement between T6 and T9 for an esophageal probe. Core temperature is then recorded every 15 minutes until reaching goal temperature, at which point temperature documentation can be spaced to hourly. After 72 hours of TH, the infant is rewarmed slowly, at no more than 0.5°C per hour to a temperature of 36.5°C to 37°C. Rewarming can be extended if the neonate becomes symptomatic with increased seizure activity, electrolyte imbalances, decreased urine output, or hypotension.

RESPIRATORY MANAGEMENT

Most neonates who qualify for TH also require mechanical ventilation after birth. Hypoxia can lead to significant persistent pulmonary hypertension (PPHN), and TH by itself has also been linked to an increase in pulmonary vascular resistance. Combined, these factors put infants undergoing TH at an increased risk for PPHN.[39,40] When caring for these infants, external stimuli should be minimized by grouping cares together when possible and keeping noise levels down. In addition, PPHN should be managed per unit protocols and TH can be discontinued if PPHN is severe and unresponsive to treatment. Blood gases should also be monitored closely for oxygenation and ventilation issues. An umbilical artery catheter is the preferred sampling method for blood gases owing to its ease of access, but if unavailable, a peripheral artery line or an arterial stick can be obtained. When infants are undergoing TH, their blood gas values will differ. At 33.5°C the pH levels will increase and Pco_2 values will seem to be lower as compared with normal body temperature values.[41] Most blood gas machines can accommodate for these variations, but the infant's temperature has to be entered to obtain the corrected results. It is important to use these corrected results when evaluating for changes in respiratory support. It is most beneficial to maintain the pH at around 7.4 and Pco_2 at around 40 mm Hg to attempt to avoid effects of overventilating or underventilating. Decreased carbon dioxide levels can cause cerebral vasoconstriction, which leads to decreased CBF and eventually ischemic infarcts and possibly seizures. Hypercapnia has the opposite effect, with increased CBF, which can exacerbate the reperfusion injury.[40,42]

FLUID MANAGEMENT

Close monitoring of electrolytes and renal function is important during TH. Alterations in fluid volumes and constituents should be made based on these values. Likewise, fluid overload should be avoided to help decrease the chance of increasing cerebral edema. Feedings should also be avoided during TH owing to the high probability of intestinal ischemia during the hypoxic insult and the unknown effects of TH on perfusion to the bowel. These 2 factors combined lead most centers to hold feedings until shortly after infants have been rewarmed.[38]

INFECTIOUS DISEASE MANAGEMENT

Hypothermia decreases immune system function and sepsis can be a cause of HIE; therefore, it is recommended that infants being treated with TH receive antibiotics for a minimum of 2 to 3 days until a blood culture sent at birth returns negative. When using gentamicin in these infants, a trough serum concentration should be obtained before giving a second dose owing to its delayed elimination half-life during TH.[43] A third-generation cephalosporin can be an alternative to gentamicin use.

FAMILY SUPPORT

Regardless of the TH protocol chosen, every effort should be made to support the families of these infants. Any time a baby is undergoing TH, expressions of stress, depression, and anxiety are commonplace for families. What families expected to be a beautiful, uncomplicated birth has become an unforeseen nightmare with a flurry of people and equipment. It is easy to overlook the parents' thoughts and feelings when health care providers are busy, but memories parents form in these first few hours after birth can last a lifetime. Taking extra time to answer questions and explain happenings can help them to process their emotions and begin to deal with the consequences their child faces from HIE.

COMPLICATIONS OF THERAPEUTIC HYPOTHERMIA

There are only a few known complications of TH. Higher incidences of bradycardia have been seen, but do not require treatment. Thrombocytopenia has also been reported and does occasionally require platelet transfusions, but was limited to the stay in the neonatal intensive care unit. These side effects were considered to be benign and the benefits of TH were shown to outweigh the risks because the rates of CP, death, and major disability were lower in treated groups.[11] Subcutaneous fat necrosis can also be a complication of TH, but is rare. It is important to reposition infants with every care time as tolerated to avoid this problem. Also, close monitoring of skin integrity is needed to diagnose any skin breakdown or subcutaneous fat necrosis as quickly as possible to avoid further damage. Finally, increased pulmonary vascular resistance can be seen with TH, so special attention should be given to monitoring respiratory status, and any signs of PPHN.[39]

FOLLOW-UP DATA

Every TH program should have a follow-up program in place to track outcomes of infants after discharge. When follow-up data are gathered, quality improvement projects can be performed based on results. The Bayley Scales of Infant and Toddler Development-III is a common tool used to assess the neurologic development of infants and children. Scoring can be done up to 42 months of age to determine if any delays exist.[44]

FUTURE RESEARCH

The field of neonatology regarding HIE is always evolving to provide the best care possible for babies affected. A handful of therapies have been examined since the inception of TH to help accomplish this goal including melatonin and erythropoietin (EPO), among others.

Melatonin is a naturally occurring hormone that helps to regulate sleep, but also has some neuroprotective properties, including its potent antioxidant, antiapoptotic, and antiinflammatory effects.[45,46] Research has been conducted on fetal sheep that demonstrates a decrease in apoptosis, inflammation, and oxidative stress within the white matter, and prevents loss of the blood–brain barrier and astrogliosis with the addition of melatonin to TH.[46,47] Likewise, in fetal pigs treated with TH and melatonin, a decrease in apoptosis was also recognized as compared with those treated with TH alone.[45] Although these studies provide some promising outcomes, they are also limited by their low power, differences between trial methods, and lack of human subjects. Further clinical trials using TH with melatonin involving neonates are warranted to determine its effectiveness.

Another hormone therapy being studied is the use of EPO with TH. EPO is a naturally produced cytokine in specialized cells in the kidneys and helps with the formation of red blood cells in the bone marrow. When oxygen levels are low in the blood perfusing the kidneys, these specialized cells are stimulated to generate and release EPO. EPO, in turn, activates the bone marrow to produce more red blood cells to increase the oxygen-carrying capacity of the blood. EPO has also been shown to demonstrate significant neuroprotective and regenerative effects in the brain. In high doses given to primates, TH combined with EPO eliminated death and moderate to severe CP. Motor function was also protected.[48]

In addition, a phase II trial of 50 neonates compared TH alone with TH with EPO. This study showed a significant decrease in brain injury in infants treated with TH and EPO. At 12 months, they exhibited significantly higher Alberta Infant Motor Scale scores than their peers treated with TH alone.[49]

Another trial involving 22 newborns with HIE treated with TH and EPO had promising results, but no control group was included, so it was impossible to determine if results were better than they would have been without EPO. However, it was concluded that high-dose EPO was safe for use in neonates with HIE. Adverse outcomes assessed were lower in this study as compared with larger trials.[50] Again, these study results are restricted by the low number of participants and differences in trial methods, but show some promising outcomes worth further study. Ultimately, more research is needed to determine if any of these therapies would be useful in the treatment of HIE, but many have promising preliminary results.

SUMMARY

TH remains an integral care piece for neonates suffering from HIE. It is crucial to recognize infants with HIE as early as possible so that TH can be initiated before the secondary energy failure stage is entered. A prompt, thorough neurologic examination should be conducted by a qualified professional as soon as HIE is suspected. Those infants qualifying for TH should then be cooled based on unit protocols. Although there is still room for research in the field of TH, the advances that have already been made have improved outcomes and changed lives for thousands of children and their families.

REFERENCES

1. Perlman JM. Brain injury in the term infant. Semin Perinatol 2004;28(6):415–24.
2. Martin JA, Hamilton BE, Ventura SJ, et al. Births: final data for 2010. Natl Vital Stat Rep 2012;61:1–72.
3. Zanelli SA, Stanley DP, Kaufman DA. Hypoxic-ischemic encephalopathy. 2014. Available at: http://emedicine.medscape.com/article/973501-overview. Accessed November 20, 2017.

4. Gunn AJ, Thoresen M. Hypothermic neuroprotection. NeuroRx 2006;3:154–69.
5. Gluckman PD, Wyatt JS, Azzopardi D, et al. Selective head cooling with mild systemic hypothermia after neonatal encephalopathy: multicentre randomised trial. Lancet 2005;365(9460):663–70.
6. Shankaran S, Laptook A, Ehrenkranz R, et al. Whole body hypothermia for neonates with hypoxic-ischemic encephalopathy. N Engl J Med 2005;353(15): 1574–84.
7. Azzopardi D, Brocklehorst P, Edwards D, et al. The TOBY Study. Whole body hypothermia for the treatment of perinatal asphyxial encephalopathy: a randomised controlled trial. BMC Pediatr 2008;8:17.
8. Sarnat HB, Sarnat MS. Neonatal encephalopathy following fetal distress. A clinical and electroencephalographic study. Arch Neurol 1976;33(10):696–705.
9. Weeke LC, Vilan A, Toet MC, et al. A comparison of the Thompson Encephalopathy score and amplitude-integrated electroencephalography in infants with perinatal asphyxia and therapeutic hypothermia. Neonatology 2017;112(1):24–9.
10. Thorsen P, Jansen-van der Weide MC, Groenendaal F, et al. The Thompson encephalopathy score and short-term outcomes in asphyxiated newborns treated with therapeutic hypothermia. Pediatr Neurol 2016;60:49–53.
11. Jacobs S, Hunt R, Tarnow-Mordi W, et al. Cooling for newborns with hypoxic ischemic encephalopathy. Cochrane Database Syst Rev 2007;4:1–45.
12. Shankaran S, Laptook A, Pappas A, et al. Effect of depth and duration of cooling on deaths in the NICU among neonates with hypoxic ischemic encephalopathy: a randomized clinical trial. JAMA 2014;312(24):2629–39.
13. Atici A, Celik Y, Gulasi S, et al. Comparison of selective head cooling therapy and whole body cooling therapy in newborns with hypoxic ischemic encephalopathy: short term results. Turk Pediatri Ars 2015;50(1):27–36.
14. Sarkar S, Barks JD, Bhagat I, et al. Effects of therapeutic hypothermia on multiorgan dysfunction in asphyxiated newborns: whole-body cooling versus selective head cooling. J Perinatol 2009;29(8):558–63.
15. Hogue N, Chakkarapani E, Liu X, et al. A comparison of cooling methods used in therapeutic hypothermia for perinatal asphyxia. Pediatrics 2010;126(1):e124–30.
16. Celik Y, Atici A, Gulasi S, et al. Comparison of selective head cooling versus whole-body cooling. Pediatr Int 2016;58(1):27–33.
17. Shankaran S, Laptook A, Wright LL, et al. Whole-body hypothermia for neonatal encephalopathy: animal observations as a basis for a randomized, controlled pilot study in term infants. Pediatrics 2002;110(2 pt 1):377–85.
18. Akisu M, Huseyinov A, Yalaz M, et al. Selective head cooling with hypothermia suppresses the generation of platelet-activating factor in cerebrospinal fluid of newborn infants with perinatal asphyxia. Prostaglandins Leukot Essent Fatty Acids 2003;69(1):45–50.
19. Merchant N, Azzopardi D. Early predictors of outcome in infants treated with hypothermia for hypoxic-ischaemic encephalopathy. Dev Med Child Neurol 2015; 57(Suppl. 3):8–16.
20. Horn A, Swingler G, Myer L, et al. Early clinical signs in neonates with hypoxic ischemic encephalopathy predict an abnormal amplitude-integrated electroencephalogram at age 6 hours. BMC Pediatr 2013;13:52.
21. Del Rio R, Ocoa C, Alarcon A, et al. Amplitude integrated electroencephalogram as a prognostic tool in neonates with hypoxic-ischemic encephalopathy: a systematic review. PLoS One 2016;11(11):e0165744.

22. Chandrasekaran M, Chaban B, Montaldo P, et al. Predictive value of amplitude-integrated EEG (aEEG) after rescue hypothermic neuroprotection for hypoxic ischemic encephalopathy: a meta-analysis. J Perinatol 2017;37(6):684–9.
23. Massaro AN, Tsuchida T, Kadom N, et al. aEEG evolution during therapeutic hypothermia and prediction of NICU outcome in encephalopathic neonates. Neonatology 2012;102(3):197–202.
24. Dix LM, van Bel F, Lemmers PMA. Monitoring cerebral oxygenation in neonates: an update. Front Pediatr 2017;5:46.
25. Gumulak R, Lucanova LC, Zibolen M. Use of near-infrared spectroscopy (NIRS) in cerebral tissue oxygenation monitoring in neonates. Biomed Pap Med Fac Univ Palacky Olomouc Czech Repub 2017;161(2):128–33.
26. Lemmers PM, Zwanenburg RJ, Benders MJ, et al. Cerebral oxygenation and brain activity after perinatal asphyxia: does hypothermia change their prognostic value? Pediatr Res 2013;74(2):180–5.
27. Goeral K, Urlesberger B, Giordano V, et al. Prediction of outcomes in neonates with hypoxic-ischemic encephalopathy II: role of amplitude-integrated electroencephalography and cerebral oxygen saturation measured by near-infrared spectroscopy. Neonatology 2017;112(3):193–202.
28. Low E, Boylan GB, Mathieson SR, et al. Cooling and seizure burden in term neonates: an observational study. Arch Dis Child Fetal Neonatal Ed 2012;97:F267–72.
29. Gillam-Krakauer M, Carter BS. Neonatal hypoxia and seizures. Pediatr Rev 2012;33:9.
30. Lynch NE, Stevenson NJ, Livingstone V, et al. The temporal characteristics of seizures in neonatal hypoxic ischemic encephalopathy treated with hypothermia. Seizure 2015;33:60–5.
31. Vanucci RC. Hypoxic-ischemic encephalopathy. Am J Perinatol 2000;17(3):113–20.
32. Rutherford MA, Pennock JM, Schwieso JE, et al. Hypoxic ischaemic encephalopathy: early magnetic resonance imaging findings and their evolution. Neuropediatrics 1995;26:183–91.
33. Rollins N, Booth T, Morriss MC, et al. Predictive value of neonatal MRI showing no or minor degrees of brain injury after hypothermia. Pediatr Neurol 2014;50(5):447–51.
34. Chilla GS, Tan CH, Xu C, et al. Diffusion weighted magnetic resonance imaging and its recent trend-a survey. Quant Imaging Med Surg 2015;5(3):407–22.
35. Van Laerhoven H, de Haan TR, Offringa M, et al. Prognostic tests in term neonates with hypoxic-ischaemic encephalopathy: a systematic review. Pediatrics 2013;102:707–11.
36. Roka A, Melinda KT, Vasarhelyi B, et al. Elevated morphine concentrations in neonates treated with morphine and prolonged hypothermia for hypoxic ischemic encephalopathy. Pediatrics 2008;121(4):e844–9.
37. Fritz HG, Holzmayr M, Walter B, et al. The effect of mild hypothermia on plasma fentanyl concentration and biotransformation in juvenile pigs. Anesth Analg 2005;100(4):996–1002.
38. Zanelli S, Buck M, Fairchild K. Physiologic and pharmacologic considerations for hypothermia therapy in neonates. J Perinatol 2011;31(6):377–86.
39. Benumof JL, Wahrenbrock EA. Dependency of hypoxic pulmonary vasoconstriction on temperature. J Appl Physiol Respir Environ Exerc Physiol 1977;42(1):56–8.

40. Wintermark P. Brain cooling for asphyxiated newborns: the impact on respiratory mechanics, oxygenation and ventilation. Can J Respir Ther 2012;48(1):13–6.
41. Groenendaal F, De Vooght KM, van Bel F. Blood gas values during hypothermia in asphyxiated term neonates. Pediatrics 2009;123(1):170–2.
42. Hansen NB, Brubakk AM, Bratlid D, et al. The effects of variations in PaCO2 on brain blood flow and cardiac output in the newborn piglet. Pediatr Res 1984; 18(11):1132–6.
43. Mark LF, Solomon A, Northington FJ, et al. Gentamicin pharmacokinetics in neonates undergoing therapeutic hypothermia. Ther Drug Monit 2013;35(2):217–22.
44. Bayley N. Bayley scales of infant and toddler development: administration manual. San Antonio (TX): Harcourt Assessment.; 2006.
45. Robertson NJ, Faulkner S, Fleiss B, et al. Melatonin augments hypothermic neuroprotection in a perinatal asphyxia model. Brain 2013;136(pt 1):90–105.
46. Yawno T, Mahen M, Li J, et al. The beneficial effects of melatonin administration following hypoxia ischemia in preterm fetal sheep. Front Cell Neurosci 2017;11: 296.
47. Yawno T, Castillo-Melendez M, Jenkin G, et al. Mechanisms of melatonin-induced protection in the brain of late gestation fetal sheep in response to hypoxia. Dev Neurosci 2012;34:543–51.
48. Traudt CM, McPherson RJ, Bauer LA, et al. Concurrent erythropoietin and hypothermia treatment improve outcomes in a term nonhuman primate model of perinatal asphyxia. Dev Neurosci 2013;35:10–1159.
49. Wu YW, Mathur AM, Change T, et al. High-dose erythropoietin and hypothermia for hypoxic-ischemic encephalopathy: a phase II trial. Pediatrics 2016;137.
50. Rogers EE, Bonifacio SL, Glass HC, et al. Erythropoietin and hypothermia for hypoxic-ischemic encephalopathy. Pediatr Neurol 2014;51(5):657–62.

APPENDIX 1: HYPOTHERMIA GUIDELINES

Guideline: Induced hypothermia for perinatal encephalopathy of infants.

Purpose: Therapeutic hypothermia to optimize neurologic outcomes in infants 35 weeks or older with perinatal encephalopathy.

Implementation of therapy will be determined after a full clinical assessment by the treating neonatologist based on the following criteria:

All of these:

- 35 weeks or greater gestation
- 1800 g or greater
- 6 hours of age or less
- Clinical encephalopathy as defined by presence of seizures, or 2 or more of the following:
  - Altered mental status such as lethargy, stupor, or coma;
  - Abnormal tone (hypotonia or flaccid);
  - Abnormal primitive reflexes (absent/weak suck, incomplete or absent Moro);
  - Decreased or no spontaneous activity;
  - Abnormal posture (distal flexion or decerebrate); and
  - Autonomic instability (constricted or unequal pupils; bradycardia or variable heart rate; periodic breathing or apnea).

Category	Moderate Encephalopathy	Severe Encephalopathy
Consciousness	Lethargic	Stupor/coma
Tone	Hypotonia (focal or general)	Flaccid
Primitive reflexes: suck, Moro	Weak, incomplete	Absent
Activity	Decreased	No activity
Posture	Distal flexion	Decerebrate
Autonomic		
Pupils Heart rate Respirations	Constricted bradycardia Periodic	Fixed; unequal Variable heart rate Apnea

With the following clinical parameters:

- Cord gas or postnatal blood gas obtained within 1 hour of life with a pH of 7.0 or less or a base deficit of 16 or greater.
- Or, if blood gas not available or marginal blood gas,[1] and suspected perinatal event,[2] then
  - Apgar score of 5 or less or less at 10 minutes, or
  - Prolonged resuscitation (ie, chest compressions, endotracheal tube/mask ventilation at 10 minutes of life).

1. Marginal blood gas is defined as pH 7.01 to 7.15 or Base deficit of 10 to 16.
2. Suspected perinatal ischemic event such as late/variable decelerations, cord prolapse, cord rupture, uterine rupture, and maternal trauma/hemorrhage/cardiorespiratory arrest.

Exclusion Criteria

- Over 6 hours of age
- Under1800 g

- Intrauterine growth restriction/small for gestational age (<10% head or length)
- Coagulopathy with active bleeding
- Persistent pulmonary hypertension requiring extracorporeal membrane oxygenation
- Major congenital abnormalities, including, but not limited to, lethal aneuploidy, abdominal wall defects, congenital heart disease, known or highly suspected metabolic disease and major brain abnormalities (including documented intracranial hemorrhage).
- Death seems to be inevitable with poor response to resuscitative measures.

Modes of Neonatal Ventilation: Breathe Deeply!

Shawn Hughes, BS, RRT-NPS, CPFT

KEYWORDS

• Neonatal • Intensive care • Respiratory distress • Ventilator • Prematurity

KEY POINTS

- The vast majority of neonates born at less than 28 weeks of gestation will require respiratory support to facilitate gas exchange.
- Clear-cut criteria on whether to initiate noninvasive or invasive ventilation are subject to interpretation and provider preference.
- Minimizing the unfavorable effects of mechanical ventilation requires an understanding of the principles of ventilation and the specific pathophysiology to which they are being applied.

INTRODUCTION

The vast majority of neonates born at less than 28 weeks of gestation will require respiratory support to facilitate gas exchange.[1] Chronic lung disease (CLD) is defined as the need for supplemental oxygen use at 36 weeks of postmenstrual age or at discharge/transfer before 36 weeks in infants who survived to 36 weeks. CLD continues to be the most frequent and serious morbidity in ventilated preterm infants today. Although the incidence of CLD has declined from the early 1970s, the incidence of CLD remains highly variable from institution to institution.

Historically, nurses and other health care providers have witnessed the sequela of mechanical ventilation, most notably from the presurfactant era, including the use of antenatal steroids, postnatal steroids, and delivery room management protocols. Uncertainty still exists regarding the best initial respiratory management strategy in terms of mode or device. Clear-cut criteria on whether to initiate noninvasive or invasive ventilation are subject to interpretation and provider preference.

The advances in ventilator technology have continued to evolve over the past 50 years. However, the most effective means of effective ventilation of the neonate continues to be a major challenge in respiratory care. The engineering advances in

---

Disclosure: The author has nothing to disclose.
NICU Respiratory Care Services, Charlotte R. Bloomberg Children's Center, Neonatal Intensive Care Unit, Johns Hopkins Hospital, 8th Floor, 1800 Orleans Street, Baltimore, MD 21287, USA
E-mail address: shughes8@jhmi.edu

Crit Care Nurs Clin N Am 30 (2018) 523–531
https://doi.org/10.1016/j.cnc.2018.07.008

the development of devices with complex capabilities have outpaced the understanding of how and when to use them optimally.[2] Early mechanical ventilators for neonates were derivations of adult ventilators and were volume cycled. Modern ventilators are designed to function with an array of patients, including adults, children, and neonates. A few manufacturers have ventilators designed specifically for the pediatric/neonatal population.

It is important that the selection of ventilator modalities be evidence-based. There is a lack of level 1 evidence to guide ventilator modalities. This is due in part to the difficulties involved in designing randomized control trials, but also individual patients may respond differently to various modalities based on their unique physiology, severity of illness, and variable susceptibility to ventilator-induced lung injury (VILI).[1] When evidence is lacking, the goal of any ventilation strategy should be to assist ventilation without causing lung injury, treating lung injury when it occurs, and facilitating adequate oxygenation while avoiding hyperventilation. A mechanical ventilator will inevitably cause some degree of lung injury even if managed optimally by health care providers. Minimizing the unfavorable effects of mechanical ventilation requires an understanding of the principles of ventilation and the specific pathophysiology to which they are being applied.

NASAL CONTINUOUS POSITIVE AIRWAY PRESSURE

There is little debate that nasal continuous positive airway pressure (nCPAP) is the preferred respiratory support in the treatment of respiratory distress syndrome (RDS) in neonates today.[3] Literature in premature infants and animal models demonstrates that positive pressure mechanical ventilation contributes to CLD and poor lung development. Hence, there is a renewed interest in nCPAP and noninvasive ventilation as a mode of therapy.

CPAP was first described over a century ago by August Ritter von Reuss and is likened to the bubble CPAP system of today. The first reported use of CPAP in neonates was not until the 1970s. Early clinical CPAP trials from this decade in preterm infants showed decreased incidence of death and the need for mechanical ventilation but increased incidence of pneumothorax.[4] Later trials in preterm infants treated prophylactically with surfactant showed a decrease in mortality, bronchopulmonary dysplasia (BPD), and air leaks.[5,6]

Currently, various interfaces and devices are employed to deliver nCPAP. This can be done through the ventilator, SiPAP specifically designed for nCPAP, or through bubble CPAP. Each mode has unique advantages and disadvantages. The goal of nCPAP is to maintain functional residual capacity (FRC), thus decreasing work of breathing and improving oxygenation and ventilation. Successful implementation and use of nCPAP require a coordinated multidisciplinary approach that includes proper sizing of equipment, monitoring of the neonate to maintain a seal, troubleshooting the nCPAP equipment, and staff education of the benefits of nCPAP. Tissue injury to the nares, nasal bridge, and columella because of improperly sized masks and prongs is a common problem. Pressure necrosis may occur if the masks and prongs are applied too tightly. This is exacerbated because of the prolonged duration of treatment that premature infants may experience. The best prevention of nasal/septal breakdown is close monitoring by the clinician. The mask or prongs must not be strapped on too tightly and sized appropriately along with the hat. One of the strategies used to prevent nasal/septal breakdown is rotation between mask and prongs at regular intervals.

A new device is the RAM cannula. Currently US Food and Drug Administration (FDA) approved as a class 1 medical device to deliver oxygen, the RAM cannula is being used as an interface to deliver nCPAP and nasal intermittent positive pressure ventilation (NIPPV). The only published evidence for neonates is a single-center observational study of 88 infants; 21 infants received noninvasive positive pressure ventilation, NIPPVV via the RAM cannula. The author concluded NIPPV via the RAM cannula was well tolerated with care guidelines.[7]

Caution must be taken when using the RAM cannula to deliver NIPPV or CPAP. In a lung simulator model, 60% to 70% of set peak inspiratory pressure (PIP) and positive end expiratory pressure (PEEP) was delivered when sized appropriately, and pressure transmission was drastically reduced, resulting in negligible pressure transmission.[8] In another lung simulator model in CPAP mode, the RAM cannula did not deliver MAP as indicated by the ventilator.[9]

BASIC MODES OF VENTILATION

Although the modern neonatal ventilator is a relatively new device in historical terms, references to ventilating infants in the medical literature has been present for centuries. Understanding the nomenclature for modes of ventilation can be confusing for nursing and other health care providers. There is no standardization of terminology in the industry, and individual manufacturers employ proprietary terminology to describe various modes. Certain ventilators set a PIP above the set PEEP level, while others set a PIP that includes the PEEP known as PEEP compensated. This can result in confusion regarding the ordered mode and parameters when setting up the ventilator.

The decision on a specific mode and ventilator strategy tends to be institution dependent and relies on a complex array of factors. Pressure control remains the most common mode of ventilation used in the neonatal intensive care unit (NICU) today. In pressure control, ventilation tidal volumes vary breath to breath. This can lead to either too large or too small tidal volumes being delivered. Tidal volume is responsible for the elimination of carbon dioxide and establishment of adequate gas exchange. In an effort to minimize lung injury, tidal volumes are usually maintained in the 4 to 6 cc/kg range. It is important to note that as lung injury evolves such as in CLD, tidal volumes of 7 to 8 cc/kg may be necessary because of a mismatch in areas of the lung being ventilated and perfused. This is known as ventilation perfusion mismatch.

CONTINUOUS MANDATORY VENTILATION

Continuous mandatory ventilation (CMV) is considered an outdated mode of neonatal ventilation. Each breath is delivered at a predetermined interval and regardless of the infant's spontaneous effort. This can cause breath stacking, asynchrony with the ventilator, increased work of breathing (WOB), and excessive lung inflation. Asynchrony with the ventilator can impact gas exchange and increase the risk for pneumothorax,[10–12] and intraventricular hemmorrage.[13] This mode is best reserved for the infant who has no spontaneous respiratory effort such as a paralyzed neonate or one under general anesthesia. CMV has largely been replaced today with assist control ventilation (AC).

ASSIST CONTROL VENTILATION

AC is a synchronous mode with a set respiratory rate, PIP, PEEP, inspired oxygen concentration, and inspiratory time (iT). All breaths are delivered at the set PIP and iT. In the event of apnea, mechanical breaths are provided at set parameters. Although this mode can be used in pressure control, it is a popular mode in a volume control mode also. The rate should be set to a minimum that will support the infant should apnea occur. AC ventilation results in a more consistent delivery of tidal volume and decreased WOB.

Caution must be taken when setting the inspiratory time so it does not produce an inflation that is either too lengthy or brief. This problem has largely been eliminated with the addition of flow cycling. Weaning in this mode is done by reducing the PIP while targeting a tidal volume of 4 to 6 cc/kg. Weaning the PIP allows the infant to take over more of the work of breathing. Weaning the respiratory rate is not necessary once the infant is maintaining a spontaneous rate as the infant is controlling the respiratory rate.

SYNCHRONIZED INTERMITTENT MANDATORY VENTILATION

Synchronized intermittent mandatory ventilation (SIMV) is an evolution from IMV in previously utilized ventilators. IMV, similar to CMV, did not sense the infant's spontaneous breaths. SIMV allows for a combination of mandatory breaths and spontaneous breaths. In SIMV, the clinician sets a respiratory rate, PIP, PEEP, iT, and oxygen concentration. All mandatory breaths are delivered at the set PIP and iT; however, the breaths are not necessarily evenly spaced. The microprocessors in modern ventilators calculate when a breath is due to be generated but may delay or deliver a breath prior to a breath being due in order to synchronize with the infant. Tidal volume varies in SIMV pressure ventilation mode. PIP should be set to deliver a tidal volume between 4 and 6 cc/kg. The tidal volume needs to be closely monitored, as changes in lung mechanics and physiology may result in a lower or higher tidal volume than desired tidal volume at the set PIP. The infant may breathe at a rate above the set rate; however, those breaths will be unsupported. Accordingly, the infant will be breathing at the set PEEP level, which may cause an increased WOB and/or tachypnea. It is therefore recommended that SIMV be used in conjunction with pressure support (PS).

PS aids the spontaneous breaths that are above the set rate. PS provides a pressure boost to augment the infant's spontaneous effort. The difference between a PS breath and a set breath is in the PS breath, the infants sets their own inspiratory time compared with a set breath, which is delivered at the set iT. There is no consensus as to what the appropriate level of PS is in neonates. It has been shown that the addition of PS increases the infant's minute volume and stabilizes the breathing pattern.[13]

PRESSURE SUPPORT VENTILATION

Pressure support ventilation (PSV) is a spontaneous mode of ventilation that supports every breath of the neonate similar to AC. A Cochrane review[14,15] was completed of available trials comparing PSV and time-cycled ventilation. Only two randomized trials were eligible for analysis involving a total of 19 patients. There were no trials addressing the impact of PSV on long-term outcomes such as CLD. Thus, it is not clear whether there is benefit to using PSV over SIMV.

In PS, a pressure level is set above PEEP in an effort to help the patient overcome the resistance of the breathing circuit and endotracheal tube, as well as support the patient's spontaneous tidal volume. When the breath is triggered, the ventilator delivers a breath to a preset pressure. Unlike AC where the breath is held for a predetermined inspiratory time, the PS breath is ended when a predetermined flow threshold is reached which is typically 15% in neonatal ventilators. At the initiation of the breath, flow rapidly enters the lungs. As the lungs fill, flow into the lungs begins to decline. When the flow into the lungs declines to 15% of the maximum flow, the breath will be ended. PSV can be used as a stand-alone mode of ventilation or in combination with other spontaneous breathing modes of ventilation such as SIMV. When used as an adjunct with SIMV, weaning is achieved by reducing the set respiratory rate while maintaining and adequate tidal volume with PS breaths. In SIMV/PS, SIMV mandatory breaths are delivered at the set Ti while during PS the infant controls the iT and the iT varies from breath to breath. PS levels should be set to achieve a tidal volume of 3.5-5 cc/kg. Adding PS to SIMV is a useful tool in a neonate who is unable to support their own spontaneous breaths. Minimum respiratory rates prior to extubation vary from institution to institution, but typically range from 10 to 20 breaths per minute. When PSV is used as a stand-alone mode of ventilation, caution must be taken for infants less than 1000 g due to very short spontaneous inspiratory times. Inspiratory time in these infants can range from approximately 0.18 to 0.23 seconds.

It is important to note that short iT in this patient population may lead to a lower than desired mean airway pressure (MAP), resulting in atelectasis, increased fi02, and increased WOB. This can be offset by increasing the set PEEP level from the typical 5 cm H_20 to 6 to 8 cm H_20. Other considerations when using PSV include endotracheal tube leak. When the endotracheal tube leak is greater than the set flow cycling percent, exhalation will not occur. It is important to set the iT in PSV appropriately to allow the breath to be time terminated when leaks are present or the neonate sighs. Some ventilators use leak compensation, which is a setting or algorithm in the ventilator that compensates for the leak. However, because of leak variability, adding or adjusting leak compensation can cause asynchrony between the ventilator and the neonate.

PRESSURE-REGULATED VOLUME CONTROL/VOLUME GUARANTEE

Volume-targeted ventilation is another popular mode used in neonatal ICUs. Pressure control ventilation has long been the standard of care in neonatal ventilation. Limiting pressure to the premature lung in an effort to reduce lung injury has been the perceived benefit of pressure ventilation. However, studies clearly demonstrate that pressure itself will not cause lung injury without the addition of excessive tidal volume. A recent meta-analysis found reduced rates of bronchopulmonary dysplasia (BPD), pneumothoraces, hypocarbia, severe cranial ultrasound pathologies, and duration of ventilation when using VTV strategies compared with pressure ventilation modes.[16]

Two popular modes using a volume ventilation strategy are volume guarantee (VG), available on Dräger ventilators, and pressure-regulated volume control (PRVC), available on Maquet ventilators. It is important for the clinician to have an awareness of how the ventilator is targeting the tidal volume. Ventilator manufacturers can target inhaled tidal volumes in volume control modes or target exhaled tidal volume. Targeting inhaled tidal volume can pose a problem in the presence of moderate-to-large endotracheal tube leaks, leading the clinician to target lower than desired tidal volumes. PRVC or VG can be used in SIMV, PSV or AC. A targeted tidal volume is set by the clinician and delivered by the ventilator at the lowest pressure necessary to inflate the lungs to the desired tidal volume. A PIP is also set, but functions as a maximum pressure limit at which the ventilator will allow the breath to be delivered.

The pressure required to inflate the neonatal lung can will vary breath to breath as lung compliance and physiology changes. This can also be seen during patient care, such as suctioning or with repositioning. As lung compliance deteriorates, the PIP required to deliver the tidal volume will increase. In an effort to protect the lungs, the ventilator will not allow large fluctuations in pressure from breath to breath. It is important to set the maximum pressure limit. The goal is to inflate the lungs at the lowest pressure while stabilizing the delivered tidal volume. In SIMV + VG mode, only the set mechanical breaths are volume targeted. Spontaneous breaths above the preset breaths in SIMV are not volume supported. SIMV + VG has been shown to be a useful tool to optimize mechanical support.[17] SIMV + VG is associated with higher work of breathing indicated by tachycardia, tachypnea, and lower SpO(2) compared with AC + VG. Volume guarantee in AC ventilation also results in more uniform tidal volume delivery with less breath-to-breath fluctuation compared with SIMV + VG.[18]

NEURALLY ADJUSTED VENTILATORY ASSIST

Neurally adjusted ventilatory assist (NAVA) is a novel mode of ventilation that involves using the electrical signal generated in the brainstem to the phrenic nerve to stimulate the diaphragm. A catheter, with 9 tiny electrodes embedded into the wall, is placed into the esophagus. The electrical signal called the EAdi signal received by the electrodes triggers the ventilator. The catheter can also be used as a feeding tube, eliminating the need for an additional tube to be placed into the esophagus. Placement of the catheter is crucial in order to obtain the proper EAdi signal. NAVA be used as either an invasive mode or noninvasive mode.

Unlike other forms of invasive ventilation, which use a pressure or flow trigger to initiate a breath and are affected by ETT leak, the benefit of using NAVA is synchronization of the ventilator with the patient's spontaneous breaths; additionally, it is not affected by tube leak. The disadvantage of NAVA is that it will not pick up a signal during apneic periods. This may limit use in extremely low birth weight infants with long periods of apnea. No large randomized controlled trials have been done to assess if NAVA has an effect on outcomes of CLD or VILI. NAVA is only available on one commercially manufactured ventilator: the SERVO-iMaquet (Maquet Critical Care, Solna, Sweden).

HIGH FREQUENCY VENTILATION

High frequency ventilation (HFV) uses tidal volumes at or less than anatomic dead space (approximately $\leq$ 1 mL/kg) and very high respiratory rates. The FDA has classified HFV devices as those that deliver a respiratory rate greater 150 breaths per minute. Yandell Henderson first described HFV in the literature in 1915 as adequate ventilation with small tidal volumes and rapid respiratory rates. In the 1950s to 1970s, Jack Emerson, Forrest Bird, and Bert Bunnell designed and tested different types of high frequency ventilators. There are at least 6 different types of high frequency ventilators used throughout the world. The ventilators deliver breaths in 1 of 3 ways: diaphragm oscillator, flow interrupter, or jet pulses.

HFV is typically described as being used in 1 of 3 ways, early intervention, proactive, or rescue. When HFV is used as early intervention, it is used a frontline therapy or within the first 4 hours of life. Proactive is typically used when predetermined guidelines are reached. Rescue is defined as failing other modes or gas exchange continues to deteriorate.

There are currently 2 main HFV devices used in the United States: the Bunnell Life Pulse jet ventilator and the 3100A High Frequency Oscillatory Ventilator. HFV allows for decoupled control of oxygenation and ventilation. Oxygenation depends upon alveolar recruitment and stabilization of those alveoli with MAP. Ventilation depends upon tidal volume rate. The Bunnell Life Pulse jet ventilator was FDA approved in 1988. Initially the jet vent was utilized to rescue infants with pulmonary interstitial emphysema (PIE) and air leaks. A multicenter randomized controlled trial in 1997 demonstrated a reduction in CLD at 36 weeks and no difference in IVH/PVL compared with CV.[19]

Other studies have demonstrated that HFJV is also an effective tool in treating MAS/PPHN. It uses small pulses of gas injected into a specially designed Life Port ETT adapter. Although inspiration on the jet is active, exhalation during HFJV is passive, relying on the natural elastic recoil of the lungs to exhale. The jet ventilator has only 3 settings, PIP, rate, and iT. For this reason, the jet ventilator must be used in conjunction with the conventional ventilator. The CV allows the addition of PEEP and Fi02. A low back up rate of 3 to 5 bpm, commonly referred to as "sighs" with a PIP and iT may also be added via the CV in the event that lung recruitment is necessary. The jet ventilator delivers breaths at a rate of 240 to 660 beats per minute (4–11 Hz). The rate commonly started on the jet vent on premature infants is 420 beats per minute with a PIP that produces adequate chest wiggle. Chest wiggle is used to assess adequacy of ventilation in HFV. A blood gas must be obtained to assess appropriate ventilation and oxygenation. Lower starting rates of the jet vent may be necessary in larger infants or infants who are experiencing gas trapping as seen in MAS, PIE or BPD. When transitioning to HFJV from CV, starting PIP should be set equal to or a few cm H_20 less than PIP on CV and again assessing chest wiggle.

As mentioned previously, a backup rate and PIP may be necessary to recruit the lung. This setting should be temporary and discontinued once the lung is recruited. If the lung needs recruitment during HFJV via sigh breaths, this means PEEP is inadequate. PEEP should be started at 7 to 8 cmH_20 if initiating HFJV. When transitioning to HFJV from CV, PEEP should be set 2 cm H_20 above CV PEEP to maintain MAP and lung recruitment. The 3100 A High Frequency Oscillatory Ventilator (HFOV) was first FDA approved in 1991 in neonates for treatment of all forms of respiratory failure. As discussed previously, in HFV, ventilation and oxygenation can be decoupled assuming a well-recruited lung. HFOV is considered active inhalation and active exhalation. The high-frequency oscillatory ventilation (HFOV) generates small tidal volumes using an oscillatory piston and diaphragm.

Animal studies suggest advantages of HFOV as compared with conventional ventilation for supporting immature or injured lungs.[20,21] Conversely, clinical trials comparing HFOV with conventional ventilation in infants with very low birth weight have yielded mixed results.[21–23] This may be because clinical trials varied widely in design, criteria for entry, the use or nonuse of exogenous surfactant, the strategy for lung recruitment, and the types of ventilators studied.

There are 4 settings in HFOV: MAP, Hertz (rate), time, and power (amplitude). In HFOV, oxygenation is controlled by a MAP setting similar to PEEP in CV and fi02. MAP recruits and stabilizes the lungs. MAP also improves oxygenation and has a minimal effect on ventilation unless the lung is overinflated or underinflated. An indicator that the MAP is too low is when the amplitude adjustments approach 3 times the MAP. The primary control of $C0_2$ is the power or amplitude setting. This produces a peak to trough swing (amplitude) across the MAP. Some institutions follow the power setting, while others follow the amplitude displayed when the power knob is adjusted. Increasing the amplitude will increase tidal volume thus increase ventilation. Conversely decreasing amplitude will have the opposite effect. Increasing amplitude can also improve oxygenation especially in atelectatic areas of the lung. Secondary control of $C0_2$ is done using the frequency or Hz. In simple terms, adjusting the Hz is actually what controls the respiratory rate of the oscillator. Adjusting the oscillator includes 1 Hz = 60 breaths per minute change and the range on the oscillator is 180 to 900 bpm (3–15 Hz). Increasing the frequency on the HFOV decreases tidal volume due to the I: E ratio being held constant at 1:2. Initial setting and management change for various disease states and are beyond the scope of this writing.

Successful HFV strategy is much like that of conventional ventilation. The clinician must have a thorough knowledge of lung mechanics and pathophysiology and understand the characteristics of the specific HFV devices. Best practice for initiating HFV is establishing criteria for initiating HFV, and applying lung protective ventilation by recruiting, stabilizing and ventilating the lung gently. Some common practice for initiating HFV is on micro-preemies that fail NCPAP, PIE, RDS, air leaks, CDH, MAS, PPHN, and pneumonia.

SUMMARY

Mechanical ventilation strategies of premature infants has changed significantly over the past 30 years. Success depends of a variety of factors, not only respiratory management related, but also overall neonatal management. There is no standardization of what is considered a failure of nCPAP requiring intubation and mechanical ventilation. Despite the renewed interest of noninvasive modes of ventilation, premature infants still require invasive ventilation. Synchronized pressure and volume ventilation modes have become a standard of care in premature infants. It is still unclear if 1 mode is superior to another. Randomized controlled trials are essential with emerging technologies such as NAVA to address the advantages of one mode of breath triggering over the other. Current data suggest the use of volume-targeted modes of ventilation over pressure-limited in premature infants. High frequency ventilation is an alternative to conventional ventilation, as either a primary mode or secondary mode when conventional ventilation fails. Although data would suggest it is not superior to pressure-limited ventilation as a primary mode; however, it may be equally effective. Overall, choosing a mode and management strategy is complicated by the lack of level one evidence.

REFERENCES

1. Stoll BJ, Hansen NI, Bell EF, et al. Neonatal outcomes of extremely preterm infants from the NICHD Neonatal Research Network. Pediatrics 2010;126(3):443–56.
2. Keszler M. Pressure support ventilation and other approaches to overcome imposed work of breathing. Neoreviews 2006;7:e226.
3. Committee on Fetus and Newborn; American Academy of Pediatrics. Respiratory support in preterm infants at birth. Pediatrics 2014;133(1):171–4.
4. Ho JJ, Subramaniam P, Henderson-Smart DJ, et al. Continuous distending pressure for respiratory distress syndrome in preterm infants. Cochrane Database Syst Rev 2002;(2):CD002271.
5. Soll RF. Prophylactic natural surfactant extract for preventing morbidity and mortality in preterm infants. Cochrane Database Syst Rev 2000;(2):CD000511.
6. Dunn PM. Dr von Reuss on continuous positive airway pressure in 1914. Arch Dis Child 1990;65:68.
7. Nzegwu NI, Mack T, DellaVentura R, et al. Systematic use of the RAM nasal cannula in the Yale-New Haven Children's Hospital Neonatal Intensive Care Unit: a quality improvement project. J Matern Fetal Neonatal Med 2015;26(2):718–21.
8. Iyer NP, Chatburn R. Evaluation of a nasal cannula in noninvasive ventilation using a lung simulator. Respir Care 2015;60(4):508–12.
9. Gerdes JS, Sivieri EM, Abbasi S. Factors influencing delivered mean airway pressure during nasal CPAP with the RAM cannula. Pediatr Pulmonol 2016;51(1):60–9.
10. Stark AR, Bascom R, Frantz ID 3rd. Muscle relaxation in mechanically ventilated infants. J Pediatr 1979;94:439–43.

11. Greenough A, Morley CJ. Pneumothorax in infants who fight ventilators. Lancet 1984;1:689.
12. Perlman JM, Goodman S, Kreusser KL, et al. Reduction in intraventricular hemorrhage by elimination of fluctuating cerebral blood-flow velocity in preterm infants with respiratory distress syndrome. N Engl J Med 1985;312:1353–7.
13. Gupta S, Sinha SK, Donn SM. The effect of two levels of pressure support ventilation on tidal volume delivery and minute ventilation in preterm infants. Arch Dis Child Fetal Neonatal Ed 2009;94(2):F80–3.
14. Schulzke SM, Pillow J, Ewald B, et al. Flow-cycled versus time-cycled synchronized ventilation for neonates. Cochrane Database Syst Rev 2010;(7):CD008246.
15. Keszler M. INSURE, infant flow, positive pressure and volume guarantee-Tell us what is best: selection of respiratory support modalities in the NICU. Early Hum Dev 2009;85:S53–6.
16. Klingenberg C, Wheeler KI, McCallion N, et al. Volume-targeted versus pressure-limited ventilation in neonates [review]. Cochrane Database Syst Rev 2017;(10):CD003666.
17. Herrera CM, Gerhardt T, Claure N, et al. Effects of volume-guaranteed synchronized intermittent mandatory ventilation in preterm infants recovering from respiratory failure. Pediatrics 2002;110(3):529–33.
18. Abubakar K, Keszler M. Effect of volume guarantee combined with assist/control vs. synchronized intermittent mandatory ventilation. J Perinatol 2005;25(10):638–42.
19. Keszler M, Modanlou HD, Brudno DS, et al. Multicenter controlled trial of high-frequency jet ventilation in preterm infants with uncomplicated respiratory distress syndrome. Pediatrics 1997;100:593–9.
20. Froese AB, McCulloch PR, Sugiura M, et al. Optimizing alveolar expansion prolongs the effectiveness of exogenous surfactant therapy in the adult rabbit. Am Rev Respir Dis 1993;148:569–77.
21. Simma B, Luz G, Trawoger R, et al. Comparison of different modes of high-frequency ventilation in surfactant-deficient rabbits. Pediatr Pulmonol 1996;22:263–70.
22. Plavka R, Kopecky P, Sebron V, et al. A prospective randomized comparison of conventional mechanical ventilation and very early high frequency oscillatory ventilation in extremely premature newborns with respiratory distress syndrome. Intensive Care Med 1999;25:68–75.
23. Moriette G, Paris-Llado J, Walti H, et al. Prospective randomized multicenter comparison of high-frequency oscillatory ventilation and conventional ventilation in preterm infants of less than 30 weeks with respiratory distress syndrome. Pediatrics 2001;107:363–72.

Neonatal Resuscitation

Neonatal Resuscitation Program 7th Edition Practice Integration

Jeanette G. Zaichkin, RN, MN, NNP-BC*

KEYWORDS

- Neonatal resuscitation • Newborn resuscitation • Cardiopulmonary resuscitation
- Neonatal Resuscitation Program (NRP) • American Academy of Pediatrics (AAP)
- American Heart Association (AHA)

KEY POINTS

- The American Academy of Pediatrics Neonatal Resuscitation Program is the national training standard in the United States for health care professionals who manage newborn resuscitation in the hospital setting.
- Preparation for every resuscitation includes assessing perinatal risk, assembling a qualified team, conducting a briefing, checking equipment, communicating with the obstetric team, and counseling parents.
- Most vigorous term and preterm newborns benefit from delayed umbilical cord clamping for 30 to 60 seconds after birth.
- The most important and effective intervention in neonatal resuscitation is ventilation of the lungs.
- Routine intubation and tracheal suction of the nonvigorous meconium-stained newborn is no longer recommended. The nonvigorous newborn should be moved to the radiant warmer for initial steps of care and evaluation.

INTRODUCTION

The Neonatal Resuscitation Program (NRP) is an evidence-based, standardized approach to resuscitation of the newborn.[1] Launched in 1987 by the American Heart Association (AHA) and the American Academy of Pediatrics (AAP), the NRP meets the education and training needs of health care professionals in the United States who

---

Disclosure Statement: The author has a contractual relationship to produce American Academy of Pediatrics/Laerdal co-branded educational materials. She is a compensated editor and consultant for the American Academy of Pediatrics/Neonatal Resuscitation Program (NRP) and she receives no financial benefit for the sale of these materials.
Positive Pressure, PLLC, Tacoma, WA 98405, USA
* 1418 S Proctor Street, Tacoma, WA 98405.
E-mail address: Jeanette.zaichkin@outlook.com

Crit Care Nurs Clin N Am 30 (2018) 533–547
https://doi.org/10.1016/j.cnc.2018.07.009
ccnursing.theclinics.com

manage newborns in the hospital setting. As of December 2017, more than 4 million health care professionals have been NRP trained or retrained and about 200,000 learners complete the NRP provider course every year.[1] In the United States, the most current resuscitation guidelines originated from the International Liaison Committee on Resuscitation consensus on science statement.[2] Based on this international consensus document, members of the AAP NRP Steering Committee and members of the AHA wrote the Guidelines for Cardiopulmonary Resuscitation and Emergency Cardiovascular Care of the Neonate, released in October 2015.[3] The *Textbook of Neonatal Resuscitation*, 7th edition,[4] and accompanying educational materials are based on these AHA/AAP guidelines and serve to translate the guidelines into clinical practice. The NRP 7th edition materials were available in Spring 2016 and required for use on January 1, 2017.[5]

This article describes the NRP Flow Diagram[4] (**Fig. 1**) and illustrates the NRP 7th edition recommendations for resuscitation by describing 5 different resuscitation scenarios, including management of persistent central cyanosis, administration of positive-pressure ventilation (PPV; including ventilation corrective steps), management of the nonvigorous meconium-stained newborn, management of a very preterm newborn, and resuscitation of a critically ill newborn including intubation, chest compressions, and medication.

PREPARING FOR NEONATAL RESUSCITATION

A well-coordinated newborn resuscitation begins before the birth. A team with the appropriate skills must be assembled and briefed, supplies and equipment must be checked, care is coordinated with the obstetric team, and parents should be informed about the plan of care.[3,4]

Assess Perinatal Risk and Assemble the Team

The answers to 4 prebirth questions assess perinatal risk.[3,4] The questions are:

- What is the expected gestational age?
- Is the amniotic fluid clear?
- How many babies are expected?
- Are there additional risk factors?

Based on this assessment of risk, the correct number of qualified team members are assembled and briefed.[3,4] The leader is identified, roles and responsibilities are assigned, and interventions for potential scenarios are planned during this preresuscitation briefing. After every resuscitation, a debriefing gives the team a safe opportunity to offer constructive suggestions to improve teamwork and performance and indicate areas that need improvement or follow-up.[3,4]

Check Supplies and Equipment

Newborn resuscitation supplies and equipment are checked for presence and function before every birth, preferably by using a standardized checklist.[3,4]

Confirm the Plan for Umbilical Cord Clamping

Obstetric providers should delay cord clamping for at least 30 to 60 seconds for vigorous term and preterm newborns with intact placental circulation.[2–4,6,7] The benefits of delayed cord clamping for term newborns include decreasing the risk of developing iron-deficiency anemia and improving developmental outcomes. Preterm newborns benefit from decreased risks for mortality, low blood pressure, blood

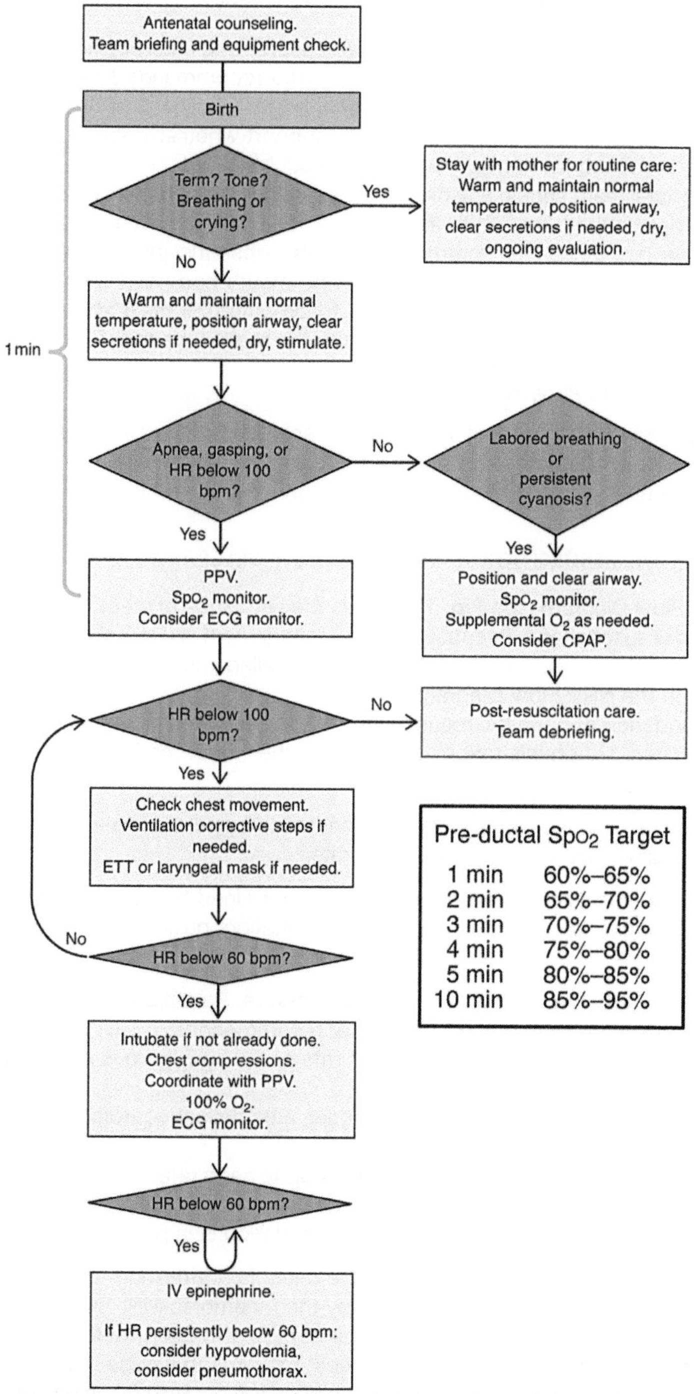

Fig. 1. NRP flow diagram. CPAP, continuous positive airway pressure; ECG, electrocardiograph; ETT, endotracheal tube; HR, heart rate; IV, intravenous; PPV, positive pressure ventilation. (*From* Weiner GM, editor. Textbook of neonatal resuscitation. 7th edition. Elk Grove Village (IL): American Academy of Pediatrics and American Heart Association; 2016. p. 244; with permission.)

transfusion after birth, brain hemorrhage, and necrotizing enterocolitis. More research is needed before delayed cord clamping can be recommended for pregnancies of twins or more, intrauterine growth restriction, or complications of placental/umbilical perfusion. There is not enough evidence to support whether delayed cord clamping should be practiced for nonvigorous newborns.[2–4,6,7]

The neonatal team should ask the obstetric provider about the plan for delayed cord clamping before the birth.[4] If the newborn is not vigorous at birth, but delayed cord clamping is not otherwise contraindicated, the obstetric provider may choose to briefly delay cord clamping while clearing the mouth and nose and stimulating the newborn. If the newborn does not begin to breathe, the cord should be clamped and cut immediately, and the baby moved to the radiant warmer.[4]

Communicate with Parents

Parents are valued members of the newborn care team. When a complex resuscitation is anticipated, or the outcome is uncertain, the neonatal medical provider shares as much information as possible and counsels parents before the birth.[4]

THE NEONATAL RESUSCITATION PROGRAM FLOW DIAGRAM

The NRP Flow Diagram (see **Fig. 1**) outlines the sequence of steps for newborn evaluation and resuscitation.[4] Because oxygen management is integral to newborn resuscitation, the preductal Spo_2 target table (also called the target saturation table) is included on the NRP Flow Diagram.[4]

The foundation of neonatal resuscitation is the inflation and ventilation of the newborn's lungs.[2–4] Administration of PPV is the most critical skill in newborn resuscitation.[3,4]

- Effective PPV inflates the lungs (demonstrated by perceptible chest movement).[4]
- Successful PPV increases the heart rate.[3,4]

When PPV is required, the next steps are determined by assessing the heart rate (**Fig. 2**).[4] Methods of assessment include auscultation, pulse oximetry, and a cardiac monitor.[3,4]

- Auscultate the apical pulse with a stethoscope. Palpation of the umbilical pulse has proven unreliable and is no longer recommended.
- If it is difficult to auscultate the heart rate of the nonvigorous infant, apply pulse oximetry.
- If pulse oximetry has an unreliable signal, attach electrocardiograph leads to the chest or limbs and use a cardiac monitor.
- A cardiac monitor provides the most accurate heart rate. Consider applying electrocardiograph leads when PPV begins. A cardiac monitor is strongly recommended for use when cardiopulmonary resuscitation is in progress.

If the heart rate is not increasing and the chest is not moving after 15 seconds of PPV, ventilation corrective steps (known by the mnemonic MR. SOPA) should begin (**Table 1**).[4] No further steps, such as chest compressions or medication, may occur until effective ventilation (evidenced by chest movement) has been administered for 30 seconds. Of course, PPV may be discontinued sooner than 30 seconds if the infant begins to breathe spontaneously and the heart rate is more than 100 bpm.[4]

After ventilation is established, the next steps of resuscitation are determined by heart rate, breathing, and oxygen saturation. It is normal for the newborn to have central cyanosis for several minutes after birth and visual assessment of oxygen

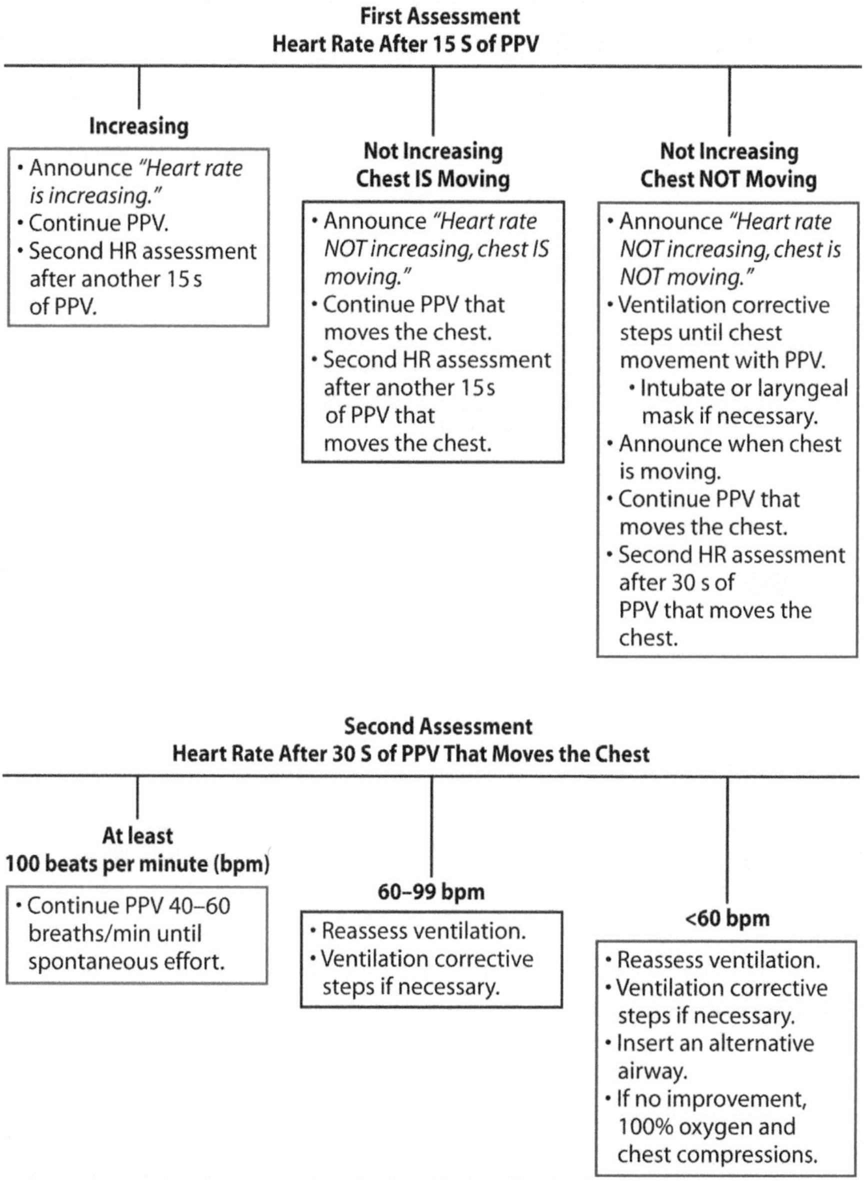

Fig. 2. Assessment of heart rate (HR). PPV, positive pressure ventilation. (*From* Weiner GM, editor. Textbook of neonatal resuscitation. 7th edition. Elk Grove Village (IL): American Academy of Pediatrics and American Heart Association; 2016. p. 84; with permission.)

saturation is not reliable.[3,4] Use of supplemental oxygen (>21%, room air) is guided by pulse oximetry and the target saturation table (see **Fig. 1**).[3,4] The goal is to prevent hypoxia and hyperoxia, both of which are injurious to the newborn. For the newborn greater than or equal to 35 weeks of gestation, PPV begins with 21% oxygen. For the newborn less than 35 weeks of gestation, PPV may begin with 21% to 30% oxygen.[3,4]

Table 1
The 6 ventilation corrective steps: MR. SOPA

	Corrective Steps	Actions
M	Mask adjustment	Reapply the mask
R	Reposition airway	Place head neutral or slightly extended
	Try PPV for several breaths and reassess chest movement	
S	Suction mouth and nose	Use a bulb syringe or suction catheter
O	Open mouth	Open the mouth and lift the jaw forward
	Try PPV for several breaths and reassess chest movement	
P	Pressure increase	Increase pressure in 5 to 10 cm H_2O increments, to maximum 40 cm H_2O for term newborn
	Try PPV for several breaths and reassess chest movement	
A	Alternative airway	Place an endotracheal tube or laryngeal mask
Try PPV and assess chest movement and breath sounds		

Abbreviation: PPV, positive pressure ventilation.

Adapted from Weiner GM, editor. Textbook of neonatal resuscitation. 7th edition. Elk Grove Village (IL): American Academy of Pediatrics and American Heart Association; 2016. p. 82; with permission.

INTEGRATION OF NEWBORN RESUSCITATION RECOMMENDATIONS INTO PRACTICE

The following scenarios illustrate selected NRP 7th edition recommendations for newborn resuscitation in the hospital delivery room. Resuscitation outside the delivery room, circumstances involving anatomic airway obstructions or congenital abnormalities, and postresuscitation care are beyond the scope of this article and described in the *Textbook of Neonatal Resuscitation, 7th edition*.[4]

A standardized equipment check is done before every birth to ensure that all supplies and equipment are present and functioning.[3,4] After each resuscitation, the team debriefs and updates parents.[4]

SCENARIO 1:
A Healthy Term Newborn is Active and Crying at Birth but Remains Cyanotic

Assess perinatal risk

See **Box 1**.

Box 1
Perinatal risk assessment for scenario 1

Gestational Age?	39 wk
Amniotic fluid clear?	Yes
	Spontaneous rupture of amniotic membranes 8 h ago
Number of babies expected?	One
Additional risk factors?	No known risk factors. Mother is healthy and has had an uncomplicated pregnancy and intrapartum period.

Assemble and brief the team

Based on the assessment of perinatal risk, newborn resuscitation is not anticipated. One team member may attend this birth and manage the newborn.[4]

Additional considerations
A full team qualified to perform all neonatal resuscitation interventions is immediately available in the hospital and the team member knows when and how to summon emergency assistance.[4]

Rapid Evaluation at Birth

- Term? Yes, the infant seems to be term, as expected.
- Muscle tone? Yes, the infant is flexed and active.
- Breathing or crying? Yes, the infant is breathing and crying without respiratory distress.

Delayed Cord Clamping and Initial Steps of Care

Umbilical cord clamping is delayed for 30 to 60 seconds. The infant is placed skin to skin on the mother's chest, with the head in a "sniffing" position to facilitate an open airway.

Ongoing Evaluation

At 3 minutes of age, the infant has no respiratory distress but still has significant persistent central cyanosis. The nurse places a pulse oximeter sensor on the infant's right hand to assess oxygen saturation using the target saturation table (see **Fig. 1**).[4] The Spo_2 is 71%, within target range for the infant's age of 3 minutes. The infant's oxygen saturation steadily increases and reaches 84% by 5 minutes of age and 93% by 10 minutes of age. At this point, the nurse decides to discontinue pulse oximetry and monitors the infant's breathing, heart rate, and temperature. To help ensure thermoregulation, the infant remains skin to skin with the mother, covered in a warm blanket. The mother offers her baby the opportunity to breastfeed.

SCENARIO 2:
A Term Newborn Requires Positive-pressure Ventilation

Assess perinatal risk
See **Box 2**.

Box 2
Perinatal risk assessment for scenario 2

Gestational Age?	39 wk
Amniotic fluid clear?	Yes
	Spontaneous rupture of amniotic membranes 10 h ago
Number of babies expected?	One
Additional risk factors?	Mother received IV narcotics 2 h ago for pain management
	Labor progressed rapidly and a vaginal birth is expected soon

Assemble and brief the team
Maternal opioid administration within 4 hours of delivery is a risk factor that requires 2 team members at the birth in case PPV is indicated.[4]

Additional considerations
A full resuscitation team is notified of the impending birth in case the newborn requires intubation or complex resuscitation.[4] The team notes that naloxone (Narcan) is no longer recommended for the newborn when maternal narcotics are suspected of decreasing the newborn's respiratory drive because of the lack of evidence evaluating the safety of naloxone use.[4,8]

Rapid Evaluation at Birth

- Term? Yes, the infant appears to be term, as expected.
- Muscle tone? No, the infant is floppy.
- Breathing or crying? No, the infant is not breathing.

Delayed cord clamping
The obstetric provider lays the infant on the mother's abdomen and begins the initial steps of newborn care. The provider suctions the mouth and nose with the bulb syringe, in anticipation of PPV and stimulates the infant briefly by drying the arms and chest with a towel. The infant does not respond by breathing; therefore, the obstetric provider clamps and cuts the cord.

Initial steps of care
The team receives the infant at the radiant warmer. The team finishes drying the infant, removes the wet linen, and positions the infant in a sniffing position to facilitate breathing. There is poor muscle tone, occasional shallow respirations and a heart rate of 70 bpm.

Positive-pressure ventilation
PPV begins within 60 seconds after birth in room air (21% oxygen). The assistant applies a pulse oximeter to the right wrist. After 15 seconds of PPV, the assistant auscultates the chest and reports a heart rate of 70 bpm, not increasing, and no chest movement with assisted breaths (see **Fig. 2**[4]). MR. SOPA ventilation corrective steps begin (see **Table 1**)[4]:

- The face mask is reapplied and the infant's head is repositioned. PPV resumes. After 4 to 5 assisted breaths, the assistant reports no chest movement.
- The infant's mouth and nose are suctioned with the bulb syringe and the mouth is opened. The mask is reapplied and PPV resumes. After 4 to 5 assisted breaths, the assistant reports no chest movement.
- The operator increases the inspiratory pressure of the assisted breaths. After a few assisted breaths, the assistant reports chest movement with PPV.

Effective PPV continues for 30 seconds. The infant's heart rate increases to 120 bpm. The infant begins to breathe spontaneously and the muscle tone improves. The oxygen saturation is within target range for the age in minutes. PPV is discontinued. The team monitors the infant's heart rate, respiratory effort, and oxygen saturation.

Ongoing evaluation
Less than 1 minute later, the infant becomes limp, the respiratory rate slows, and heart rate decreases to 80 bpm. The team resumes PPV. In response to effective ventilation, the infant's heart rate increases to more than 100 bpm and breathes spontaneously at a rate of about 30 breaths/min. The team inserts an orogastric tube to decompress the stomach and resumes PPV at a rate that sustains the heart rate at greater than 100 bpm. The neonatal team receives the infant in the nursey for further evaluation and continues respiratory support until the infant breathes effectively on his own.

SCENARIO 3:
A Newborn has Meconium-stained Amniotic Fluid and Remains Apneic after the Initial Steps of Care

Assess perinatal risk
See **Box 3**.

Box 3
Perinatal risk assessment for scenario 3

Gestational Age?	41 wk
Amniotic fluid clear?	No, the amniotic fluid is meconium stained Spontaneous rupture of amniotic membranes 2 h ago
Number of babies expected?	One
Additional risk factors?	Mother has chronic hypertension Mother is febrile Fetal heart rate has late decelerations Labor is progressing quickly and a vaginal birth is expected Estimated fetal weight is approximately 2500 g (5 lbs, 8 oz)

Assemble and brief the team

Meconium-stained amniotic fluid (MSAF) is a perinatal risk factor that increases the possibility of a compromised newborn.[2–4] If MSAF is the sole risk factor, 2 team members may attend the birth and someone with intubation skills should be identified and immediately available.[4,9] However, this scenario presents risk factors in addition to MSAF and requires a team at the birth capable of performing a complex resuscitation.[4]

Additional considerations

In the past, a nonvigorous newborn with MSAF was immediately intubated and the trachea was suctioned in an attempt to prevent the newborn from developing meconium aspiration syndrome.[2,3,4,8] Although more research is needed, there is insufficient evidence to support this practice.[2,3,4] Guidelines now recommend that routine tracheal suction not be performed for nonvigorous meconium-stained newborns. Instead, the nonvigorous meconium-stained newborn should receive the same resuscitation steps as newborns with clear amniotic fluid.[2,3,4,9]

The resuscitation team discusses the plan for delayed cord clamping with the obstetric provider before the birth.

Rapid Evaluation at Birth

- Term? The newborn is small, but features are congruent with term gestation.
- Muscle tone? No, the newborn is limp.
- Breathing or crying? No, the newborn is apneic.

Delayed cord clamping

The obstetric provider wraps the newborn in a warm towel and assesses muscle tone and respiratory effort. The newborn remains limp and apneic. The obstetric provider immediately clamps and cuts the umbilical cord.

Initial steps of care

The team receives the newborn at the radiant warmer. The infant's mouth and nose are suctioned. The infant is dried and the wet linen is removed. The baby is positioned in a sniffing position and gently stimulated to breathe, but remains limp and apneic.

Positive-pressure ventilation

PPV begins within 60 seconds after birth in room air (21% oxygen). A team member applies a pulse oximeter to the right hand. After 15 seconds of PPV, the assistant auscultates the chest and reports a heart rate of 80 bpm, not increasing, and no chest movement with assisted breaths. MR. SOPA ventilation corrective steps begin (see **Table 1**)[4]:

- The face mask is reapplied and the infant's head is repositioned. PPV resumes. After 4 to 5 assisted breaths, the assistant reports no chest movement.
- The infant's mouth and nose are suctioned with the bulb syringe and the mouth is opened. The mask is reapplied and PPV resumes. After 4 to 5 assisted breaths, the assistant reports chest movement.

PPV continues for 30 seconds. The infant's heart rate increases to 120 bpm and the infant begins to breathe spontaneously with an improvement in muscle tone.

Continuous positive airway pressure
The infant has labored, grunting respirations at a rate of 40 breaths/min. The team inserts an orogastric tube to decompress the stomach and applies continuous positive airway pressure (CPAP) at a pressure of 5 cm H_2O to help keep the airway open between breaths and ease the work of breathing.

Oxygen management
Pulse oximetry indicates that the oxygen saturation is lower than the target range for the age in minutes; therefore, the oxygen concentration is increased from 21% to 30% and the oxygen saturation increases to 78% at 4 minutes of age.

Ongoing evaluation
The newborn's vital signs are within normal limits. CPAP is in place and 30% oxygen is maintaining oxygen saturation within the target range. The infant is transported to the nursery and admitted for care.

SCENARIO 4:
Newborn Less than 32 Weeks of Gestation Requires Thermoregulation Strategies, Oxygen Management, and Continuous Positive Airway Pressure

Assess perinatal risk
See **Box 4**.

Box 4
Perinatal risk assessment for scenario 4

Gestational Age?	30 wk
Amniotic fluid clear?	Yes
Number of babies expected?	One
Additional risk factors?	No additional risk factors known. The etiology of preterm labor is unknown. The expectant mother received corticosteroids 3 d ago when she presented in the antepartum unit at high risk for preterm birth. A vaginal birth is expected.

Assemble and brief the team
A preterm infant is at considerable risk for requiring resuscitation; therefore, a team with full resuscitation skills is assembled and briefed.[4]

Additional considerations
Because the newborn is less than 32 weeks of gestation, the team uses thermoregulation strategies including increasing the room temperature to 74°F to 77°F, using a

hat, using a temperature sensor to avoid overheating or hypothermia, a thermal mattress, and a polyethylene wrap/bag.[3,4]

The lungs of a preterm infant are immature and may be difficult to ventilate. This expectant mother received corticosteroids to mature the preterm infant's lungs and improve the outcome.[10] To help keep the infant's lungs inflated between breaths, the team will use a resuscitation device that delivers positive end-expiratory pressure, such as the T-piece resuscitator, and use the lowest possible inflation pressure to avoid injury.[3,4] The use of CPAP may avoid the need for intubation and facilitate breathing if respirations are labored or oxygen saturation is below the target range despite use of supplemental oxygen.[4]

A preterm infant's heart rate may be difficult to auscultate and pulse oximetry may not display a reliable signal; therefore, a cardiac monitor offers the most accurate assessment of this newborn's heart rate.[4]

To decrease the risk of brain hemorrhage in an infant of less than 32 weeks of gestation, the team will handle the infant with care, avoid positioning the legs higher than the head, avoid higher than necessary inflation pressure during PPV, and avoid rapid infusion of intravenous fluids.[4]

Rapid Evaluation at Birth

- Term? No. The newborn has features congruent with 30 weeks of gestation.
- Muscle tone? Yes, the newborn has muscle tone appropriate for her gestational age.
- Breathing or crying? Yes, the newborn has a weak cry.

Delayed cord clamping

The obstetric provider covers the newborn in polyethylene wrap and places a warm blanket on top. The obstetric provider and a member of the neonatal team monitor the newborn's breathing and heart rate while delaying cord clamping for about 30 seconds. The umbilical cord is clamped and cut.

Initial steps of care

The infant is placed on the thermal mattress under the radiant warmer and carefully placed in the sniffing position. The infant has few oral secretions and is breathing, so the mouth and nose are not suctioned at this time. No drying is done but the polyethylene wrap covers the infant from the neck down. A hat is placed on the head and the temperature sensor and pulse oximeter are applied. Limb leads are connected to a cardiac monitor. The infant is breathing, heart rate is 140 bpm, and oxygen saturation is 65% at 2 minutes of age.

Positive-pressure ventilation

PPV is not indicated. Intubation is avoided.

Continuous positive airway pressure

Because the newborn has labored respirations, an orogastric tube is placed to decompress the stomach and CPAP is administered at 5 cm H_2O at 30% oxygen.

Oxygen management

The oxygen saturation is 77% at 3 minutes of age and the oxygen concentration is decreased to 25%.

Ongoing evaluation

At 5 minutes of age, the newborn's heart rate is 140 bpm and the respiratory rate is 60 breaths/min. The infant is receiving CPAP at 5 cm H_2O and 25% oxygen. Oxygen saturation is 84%, within target range and temperature is 36.5°C. The team moves the infant to the intensive care nursery for continued care and assessment.

SCENARIO 5:
Term Newborn Requires Intubation, Chest Compressions, and Medication

Assess perinatal risk
See **Box 5**.

Box 5
Perinatal risk assessment for Scenario 5

Gestational Age?	38 wk
Amniotic fluid clear?	Yes, spontaneous rupture of membranes about 6 minutes ago
Number of babies expected?	One
Additional risk factors?	Emergency cesarean delivery for umbilical cord prolapse with fetal bradycardia (fetal heart rate = 60–70 bpm for past 7 min) Maternal general anesthesia

Assemble and brief the team
This infant is at high risk for complex resuscitation. A full team with skills including intubation and umbilical venous catheter placement is assembled and briefed.[4]

Additional considerations
An infant that requires complex resuscitation may develop signs of hypoxic-ischemic encephalopathy.[11] Therapeutic hypothermia has been shown to decrease risk of death and improve neurologic outcomes in term and late preterm infants with moderate to severe hypoxic-ischemic encephalopathy.[12] The team will maintain the infant's temperature within target range during resuscitation and further evaluate the newborn for eligibility for therapeutic hypothermia during postresuscitation care.

Rapid Evaluation at Birth

- Term? Yes, the infant appears to be term, as expected.
- Muscle tone? No, the infant is limp.
- Breathing or crying? No, the infant is not breathing.

Delayed cord clamping
The obstetric provider quickly wraps the newborn in a warm towel. The newborn remains limp and apneic. The obstetric provider immediately clamps and cuts the umbilical cord.

Initial steps of care
The team receives the newborn at the radiant warmer. The infant's mouth and nose are suctioned in anticipation of PPV. The infant is dried, and wet linen is removed and the infant is positioned in the sniffing position. Breathing is assessed, but the infant remains limp and apneic.

Positive-pressure ventilation
PPV begins within 60 seconds of birth. The pulse oximeter is applied to the right wrist but displays no signal owing to the newborn's low heart rate and poor perfusion. The team anticipates a complex and prolonged resuscitation; therefore, electrocardiograph leads are applied to the chest and a cardiac monitor displays an accurate heart

rate. A temperature sensor is applied to the infant's skin to maintain the infant's temperature within target range.

After 15 seconds of PPV, the cardiac monitor displays a heart rate of 40 bpm and not increasing, and the assistant reports no chest movement with assisted breaths. MR. SOPA ventilation corrective steps begin (see **Table 1**)[4]:

- The face mask is reapplied, and the infant's head is repositioned and PPV resumes. After 4 to 5 assisted breaths, the assistant reports chest movement.

PPV that inflates the lungs (indicated by chest movement) continues for 30 seconds; however, the heart rate remains at about 50 bpm.

Intubation

The newborn is intubated. The assistant confirms bilateral breath sounds, chest movement, and the correct depth of tube insertion. The tube is secured. The CO_2 detector does not indicate carbon dioxide exchange owing to the infant's poor perfusion. The newborn receives 30 more seconds of PPV via the endotracheal tube, but the heart rate remains at less than 60 bpm.

Chest compressions

The oxygen concentration is increased to 100%. Compressions are coordinated with ventilations and delivered at a ratio of 3 compressions to 1 ventilation. After 60 seconds, compressions are paused, and the heart rate is assessed. The cardiac monitor displays a heart rate of about 40 bpm. Cardiopulmonary resuscitation resumes.

Vascular access

A qualified team member inserts an emergency umbilical venous catheter.

Medication administration

Epinephrine (1 mg/10 mL) is indicated.[3,4] One intratracheal dose of epinephrine may be given while vascular access is being established; however, the endotracheal route is less effective than the intravenous and intraosseous routes.[3,4] The neonatal medical provider and the medication nurse use closed loop communication to order and safely administer epinephrine via the umbilical venous catheter.[4]

Ongoing evaluation

Sixty seconds after epinephrine administration, compressions are paused and the heart rate is assessed. The cardiac monitor displays a heart rate of 52 bpm. Compressions and ventilation continue. The team ensures that 100% oxygen is in use and confirms equal bilateral breath sounds and chest movement with ventilation. The infant is pale and has weak pulses. The team considers the history of umbilical cord prolapse and suspects hypovolemic shock.

Volume administration

Emergency volume expansion (10 mL/kg) is indicated.[3,4] The newborn's estimated weight is 3 kg. The team administers 30 mL of normal saline over 5 to 10 minutes via the umbilical venous catheter.[3,4]

Ongoing evaluation

As volume is administered, the newborn's heart rate gradually increases. Compressions are stopped when the heart rate is greater than 60 bpm and assisted ventilation continues. As the heart rate increases to 110 bpm, the CO_2 detector turns yellow, indicating exhaled CO_2. The pulse oximeter indicates an oxygen saturation of 72% and increasing. The team gradually weans the oxygen from 100% to 50% to maintain the oxygen saturation within target range (≤95% at 10 minutes of age[4]). The newborn is limp and has no spontaneous respirations. The temperature is 36.7°C, which is within target range. The newborn is moved to the intensive care nursery for further evaluation and to determine eligibility for therapeutic hypothermia.

SUMMARY

The NRP has been very successful in meeting the learning needs of health care professionals who manage the newborn in the hospital setting.[1] The most current guidelines for neonatal resuscitation were released by the AAP and the AHA in October 2015.[3] The NRP 7th edition materials launched in Spring 2016, and were required for use on January 1, 2017.[5]

The quality of newborn resuscitation has lifelong impact on an infant's health and future development. Any health care professional who manages newborn care must stay current with evidence-based practice, proficient with hands-on skills, and capable of modeling behavioral skills that optimize teamwork and communication. Continuous professional development contributes to the best possible resuscitation performance and neonatal outcome.

ACKNOWLEDGMENTS

I would like to acknowledge the assistance of Rachel DePauw, MPH, Manager, Neonatal Resuscitation Program, Life Support Initiatives, American Academy of Pediatrics for her consultation during preparation of this article.

REFERENCES

1. American Academy of Pediatrics (AAP). Neonatal resuscitation program: history. Available at: https://www.aap.org/en-us/continuing-medical-education/life-support/NRP/Pages/History.aspx. Accessed December 20, 2017.
2. Perlman JM, Wyllie J, Kattwinkel J, et al. Part 7: neonatal resuscitation: 2015 international consensus on cardiopulmonary resuscitation and emergency cardiovascular care science with treatment recommendations. Circulation 2015;132(16 suppl 1):S204–41. Available at: https://doi.org/10.1161/CIR.0000000000000302. Accessed December 14, 2017.
3. Wyckoff MH, Aziz K, Escobedo MB, et al. Part 13: neonatal resuscitation: 2015 American Heart Association guidelines update for cardiopulmonary resuscitation and emergency cardiovascular care. Circulation 2015;132(18 suppl 2):S543–60. Available at: http://circ.ahajournals.org/content/132/18_suppl_2/S543.full https://doi.org/10.1161/CIR.0000000000000267. Accessed December 14, 2017.
4. Weiner GM, editor. Textbook of neonatal resuscitation. 7th edition. Elk Grove Village (IL): American Academy of Pediatrics and American Heart Association; 2016.
5. American Academy of Pediatrics (AAP). Summary of the revised neonatal resuscitation guidelines. NRP Instructor Update 2015;24(2):1–11. Available at: https://www.aap.org/en-us/Documents/nrp_newsletter_2015_fallwinter.pdf. Accessed December 20, 2017.
6. Committee on Obstetric Practice. Committee opinion no. 684: delayed umbilical cord clamping after birth. Obstet Gynecol 2017;129:e5–10. Available at: https://www.acog.org/-/media/Committee-Opinions/Committee-on-Obstetric-Practice/co684.pdf?dmc=1&ts=20171215T0418479380. Accessed December 14, 2017.

7. Delayed umbilical cord clamping after birth. Pediatrics 2017;139(6):e20170957. Available at: http://pediatrics.aappublications.org/content/pediatrics/early/2017/05/25/peds.2017-0957.full.pdf. Accessed December 14, 2017.
8. Kattwinkel J, Perlman JM, Aziz K, et al. Part 15: neonatal resuscitation: 2010 American Heart Association guidelines for cardiopulmonary resuscitation and emergency cardiovascular care. Circulation 2010;122(suppl 3):S909–19. Available at: http://circ.ahajournals.org/cgi/content/full/122/18_suppl_3/S639. Accessed December 14, 2017.
9. Delivery of a newborn with meconium-stained amniotic fluid. Committee opinion No. 689. American College of Obstetricians and Gynecologists. Obstet Gynecol 2017;129:e33–4. Available at: https://www.acog.org/Resources-And-Publications/Committee-Opinions/Committee-on-Obstetric-Practice/Delivery-of-a-Newborn-With-Meconium-Stained-Amniotic-Fluid. Accessed December 15, 2017.
10. Antenatal corticosteroid therapy for fetal maturation. Committee opinion No. 713. American College of Obstetricians and Gynecologists. Obstet Gynecol 2017;130:e102–9. Available at: https://www.acog.org/Resources-And-Publications/Committee-Opinions/Committee-on-Obstetric-Practice/Antenatal-Corticosteroid-Therapy-for-Fetal-Maturation. Accessed December 20, 2017.
11. Rainaldi MA, Perlman JM. Pathophysiology of birth asphyxia. Clin Perinatol 2016;43(3):409–22.
12. Committee on Fetus and Newborn. Hypothermia and neonatal encephalopathy. Pediatrics 2014;133(6):1146–50. Available at: www.pediatrics.org/cgi/doi/10.1542/peds.2014-0899 doi:10.1542/peds.2014-0899. Accessed December 20, 2017.

Neonatal Pain

Perceptions and Current Practice

Mallory Perry, BSN, MS, RN, CPN[a], Zewen Tan[b], Jie Chen, BS, MSN, RN[a], Tessa Weidig[a], Wanli Xu, BS, MS, RN[a], Xiaomei S. Cong, PhD, RN[c,*]

KEYWORDS

• Pain • Neonatal care • Nonpharmacologic intervention • Pharmacologic intervention • Barriers

KEY POINTS

- Neonates are more hypersensitive to painful stimuli, due to their immature nervous system and decreased inhibition of nociceptive pain.
- Poorly treated pain in neonates may lead to lifelong consequences, including altered neurobehavioral development.
- There are more than 40 pain assessment scales in the neonate population, which may standardize assessment of pain although also provide confusion among providers.
- Nonpharmacologic and pharmacologic interventions should be used in conjunction with each other to provide a synergistic effect of pain analgesia.
- Barriers to properly managing neonate's pain include lack of time, knowledge, and influx or distrust of assessment tools and disagreement between providers.

INTRODUCTION

The knowledge of pain in neonates has increased dramatically in the past 3 decades. It has been well established that newborns can detect, process, and respond to painful stimuli.[1] Preterm infants are even more hypersensitive to pain and at greater risk for pain due to immature pain inhibition mechanisms at birth.[2] Excessive, prolonged painful events in the neonate causes adverse physiologic effects in all major organ

Disclosure Statement: This research was supported by the National Institute of Nursing Research of the National Institute of Health (R01NR016928, PI: X. Cong) and Jonas Philanthropies, Graduate Assistance in Areas of National Need, The Eastern Nursing Research Society and the Council for the Advancement of Nursing Science (PI: M. Perry).
[a] School of Nursing, University of Connecticut, 231 Glenbrook Road, Unit 4026, Storrs, CT 06269, USA; [b] Department of Molecular and Cell Biology, University of Connecticut, 91 North Eagleville Road, Unit 3125, Storrs, CT 06269-3125, USA; [c] Center for Advancement in Managing Pain, School of Nursing, University of Connecticut, 231 Glenbrook Road, Unit 4026, Storrs, CT 06269, USA
* Corresponding author.
E-mail address: xiaomei.cong@uconn.edu

Crit Care Nurs Clin N Am 30 (2018) 549–561
https://doi.org/10.1016/j.cnc.2018.07.013
0899-5885/18/
ccnursing.theclinics.com

systems, which can be life threatening and have long-term effects.[3] Interventions to alleviate neonatal pain, however, remain inadequate and inconsistently applied. Only half of the painful procedures performed in neonates were with ANALGESIA, with a wide variation in pain management practice among facilities and areas.[4] Gaps exist in knowledge, evidence, and practice in neonatal pain assessment and management, which may lead to challenges in managing the pain. The purpose of this article is to address gaps and provide a review of clinical recommendations of pain management from a historical and developmental perspective of neonatal pain.

MYSTERIES ABOUT NEONATAL PAIN

Although the field has seen many innovations, research on neonatal pain has been lacking. In 2015, an Oxford research team found evidence that babies experience pain similarly to adults.[5] MRI scans of 10 infants and adults provided a painful stimulus were compared. Results revealed that 18 of 20 brain regions active in adults experiencing pain were also active in newborns. Moreover, infants' brains showed the same level of response as adults' when exposed to a stimulus one-fourth as strong.[5] These results directly contradict the popular belief that neonates are incapable of perceiving pain.[6] Several underlying hypotheses can explain this misunderstanding. Neonates were believed incapable of interpreting pain due to their inability to create memories.[1] Combined with fears of the side effects of anesthesia, neonatal physicians performed surgeries, such as circumcision, without analgesia until the 1990s.[7] As the Oxford research results suggest, infants do feel pain and experience it more intensely than adults. The implications of this on neonatal development is staggering, considering the logistics of the neonatal ICU (NICU). Annually, 15 million premature babies are born worldwide and each may experience 300 painful surgeries during their hospitalization.[6,8] Thus, it is vital that repeated stress and insults be addressed.[4]

DEVELOPMENTAL ASPECTS OF NEONATAL PAIN

Whether or not full-term and preterm newborns have the required anatomy and physiology to sense pain contributed to the mystery. A neonate's ability to sense pain occurs with key neurodevelopment. The first step of pain sensation involves nociceptors, the nerve endings that signal pain. Cells surrounding nociceptors release pain-signaling chemicals that respond to painful stimuli.[9] In the presence of painful stimuli, a nociceptor transforms the painful signal into an impulse, propagating along an aggregation of neurons to the dorsal horn, where sensory information is received.[10] At this point, the impulse separates: one impulse returns to the initial site of pain to set off a reflexive reaction and the other reaches the thalamus. The thalamus localizes the pain of the stimuli. The brain is now equipped with information on the pain and how it can be prevented.[11]

Each stage of the nociceptive pain pathway develops at different times. At 7 weeks' gestation, nociceptive nerve endings begin to develop circumorally. Nociceptive development is complete at 20 weeks around body linings and the extremities.[12] Without any link to the spinal column, however, the nociceptor signals are not functional and are of limited use. The pathway between the nociceptive nerve endings and dorsal horn begins in week 13 and is functional by week 30.[13] With this pathway, the fetus is able to reflexively withdraw from painful stimuli but does not possess the cognitive capacity to process information regarding the pain or its source. Cortical pain perception develops after week 24 of gestation, when the thalamic track completes its connection to the dorsal horn. In short, a neonate is able to localize the pain and make reflexive movements to try to avoid it after week 24, thus completing the nociceptive pain pathway.

Another important component of the pain pathway is the myelin sheath and its role in pain modulation. The myelin sheath works as an electrical insulator, increasing the speed of a signal from the peripheral to central nervous system. Myelination develops after 25 weeks of gestation and is complete by week 37.[14] It was previously believed that unmyelinated axons were unable or too slow to transfer electrical impulses. Recent consensus is that unmyelinated neurons are fully capable of transferring a signal, although at a slower rate.[15] Pain modulation is also critical in the management of pain. Descending signal pathways protrude into the dorsal horn where pain transmission is believed halted by the release of endogenous opioids or the activation of the inhibitory pathways. Both of these mechanisms are much more prevalent in the adult than the neonate.[16] Thus, preterm infants may actually have a 30% to 50% lower pain threshold than adults and a lower pain tolerance than older children.[17] Therefore, unrelieved and repetitive painful events can result in adverse physiologic effects in all major organ systems, including brain structure. These can be life threatening and have long-term cumulative effects, including altered neurobehavioral development.[6,17]

NEONATAL PAIN ASSESSMENT

Pain assessment in neonates is notoriously difficult because of their physical, cognitive, and behavioral development. The use of pain assessment scales provides consistency between nurses and other clinicians and provides an accurate measure for the presence of pain, stress, or discomfort. These scales not only quantify pain but also can provide an accurate depiction of the effect of nonpharmacologic and pharmacologic management interventions on a neonate's pain.

It is crucial to identity any potential source of pain to facilitate pain assessment.[18] Nurses should be aware that even simple procedures and daily care, such as routine heel sticks or tape removal, can be painful and stressful and can result in altered pain perception and development in the future.[4] Recent evidence has supported that prolonged exposure to painful/stressful events are detrimental to the immature nervous system and influence the early programming of neuroimmune system in this vulnerable population.[6,19] The majority of existing instruments focused on measuring the short-term acute pain based on physiologic and behavioral cues. Few instruments are available, however, to measure persistent pain/stress in preterm infants. A recently developed tool, the Accumulated Pain/Stressor Scale,[20] could serve as an assessment scale to measure severity and acuity levels of painful/stressful procedures that hospitalized neonates undergo during a certain period of time.

Cong and colleagues[18] summarized the characteristics of many of these scales. **Table 1** summarizes several commonly used neonatal pain assessment scales. Based on their psychometric properties and purpose of usage, the Neonatal Facial Coding System (NFCS)[21]; Neonatal Pain, Agitation, and Sedation Scale (N-PASS)[22]; COMFORTneo scale[23]; Neonatal Infant Pain Scale (NIPS)[24]; and Face, Legs, Activity, Cry, and Consolability (FLACC) scale[25] are recommended for daily pain assessment. The Premature Infant Pain Profile Revised–(PIPP-R) (for neonates)[26] is recommended for pain measurement in research studies (see **Table 1**). Pain assessment should take place routinely, while the frequency of assessment is consistent with the goal of treatment.[27]

Biopsychometric approaches to pain assessment include heart rate variability,[27] skin conductance measurements,[28] and brain-oriented techniques, including

Table 1
Summary of recommended pain assessment scales for neonates

Instrument	Items/Score Range	Clinical Utility	Reliability/Validity
NFCS (Grunau & Craig,[21] 1987)	9 items: brow bulge, eye squeeze, nasolabial furrow, open lips, stretch mouth (vertical), stretch mouth (horizontal), lip purse, taut tongue, chin quiver Score: 0–9 (full-term); 0–10 (preterm)	Procedural pain; preterm, full-term	InterRR: 0.88 IntraRR: 0.83 Face, content, and construct validity: yes
FLACC (Merkel et al,[67] 1997)	5 items: face, legs, activity, cry, and consolability Score: 0–10	Postoperative pain; preverbal/ nonverbal children <7 y old	InterRR: 0.94 Content and construct validity: yes
COMFORTneo—modified from the COMFORT behavior scale (van Dijk et al,[23] 2009)	7 items: alertness, calmness/agitation, respiratory response (in mechanically ventilated children), crying (in spontaneously breathing children), body movement, facial tension, (body) muscle tone Score: 6–30	Prolonged pain Sedation level; preterm, full-term 24–42 wk GA	InterRR: 0.79 Internal consistency: 0.84–0.88 Concurrent validity: yes
NIPS (Lawrence et al,[24] 1993)	6 items: 5 behavioral items (facial expression, cry, arms, legs, and state of arousal) and 1 physiologic item (breathing pattern) Score: 0–7	Procedural pain, postoperative pain; preterm, full-term 26–47 wk GA	InterRR: 0.92–0.97 Internal consistency: 0.87–0.95 Concurrent validity: 0.53–0.84
N-PASS (Hummel et al,[22] 2008)	5 items: 4 behavioral items (crying/irritability, behavior/state, facial expression, extremities/tone, and 1 physiologic item (vital signs: heart rate, RR, BP, SaO_2) Score: 0–10	Ongoing pain (ventilation sedation level), procedural pain, postoperative pain, preterm, full-term 23–40 wk GA	Internal consistency: 0.85–0.95 InterRR: 0.88–0.93 Test-retest reliability: 0.87
PIPP (Stevens et al,[68] 1996) PIPP-R (Stevens et al,[26] 2014)	7 items: 3 behavioral items (brow bulge, eye squeeze, and nasolabial furrow), 2 physiologic items (heart rate and oxygen saturation), and 2 contextual items (gestational age and behavioral state) Score: 0–18 (full-term); 21 (preterm)	Procedural pain, postoperative pain; preterm, full-term 28–42 wk GA The most commonly used tools in research studies.	InterRR: 0.93–0.96 IntraRR: 0.94–0.98 Content and construct validity: yes

Abbreviations: BP, blood pressure; GA, gestational age; InterRR, inter-rater reliability; IntraRR, intrarater reliability; PIPP, Premature Infant Pain Profile; RR, respiratory rate; SaO2, oxygen saturation.

electroencephalography, near-infrared spectroscopy, and MRI.[29] These technologies make it possible to improve the accuracy of pain measurement in neonates, to provide clinicians with more variety of interventions and better decision making of pain management. Further research is needed to integrate these technologies into routine pain assessment in neonates.

NEONATAL PAIN MANAGEMENT: PREVENTION AND NONPHARMACOLOGIC INTERVENTIONS

Painful/stressful procedures, the total amount and duration of noxious stimuli to which the infant is exposed, must be limited to those absolutely necessary in diagnostic or therapeutic management.[30] Nonpharmacologic interventions are valuable strategies that can reduce neonatal pain directly by blocking nociceptive transduction/transmission or by activation of descending inhibitory pathways. Noninvasive techniques, such as sweet-tasting substances, kangaroo care (KC), breast milk and breastfeeding, nonnutritive sucking (NNS), swaddling, and facilitated tucking (FT), have been shown effective in soothing infants undergoing painful/stressful procedures (**Table 2**).

The administration of sucrose to neonates has been a well-researched area. A single dose of sucrose was found effective and safe for alleviating procedural pain in neonates.[30,31] The exact analgesic mechanism of sucrose on infant pain is not entirely understood.[31,32] Several animal studies have been conducted, although a main supporting hypothesis for sucrose efficacy is through activation of endogenous opioids. In activating endogenous opioids, an antinociceptive response ensues thus attenuating nociceptive signals at the dorsal horn level.[33] Evidence is still limited, however, regarding the efficacy and safety (eg, long-term neurobehavioral outcomes) of repeated use of sucrose across repeated procedural pain for neonates. Daily repeated use of sucrose (eg, >10 doses/d) in young preterm infants (eg, <31 weeks' gestational age) may lead to poor neurologic development.[31]

KC is skin-to-skin contact between an infant and parent. KC has been shown to alleviate both physiologic and behavioral responses in neonates during painful procedures.[34,35] KC works as an analgesic intervention through multisensory stimulations, including emotional, tactile, proprioceptive, vestibular, olfactory, auditory, visual, and thermal stimulations in a unique interactive style. Various durations of KC have been found effective in reducing pain in neonates when KC is provided for 10 minutes to 15 minutes,[36] 30 minutes, 80 minutes,[34,37] or 3 hours[38] before and through the procedural pain. In addition to reducing behavioral and physiologic pain responses, studies have shown that hormonal markers, including cortisol, β-endorphin, and oxytocin levels, changed in infants when receive KC,[34,39] which may explain the endogenous analgesic effect of KC in neonates.

NNS is the introduction of an oral stimulant, such as pacifier or nipple, without providing nutrition. In neonates, NNS can be used with or without the addition of sucrose, both of which have individual benefits. In the absence of sucrose, NNS remains a beneficial nonpharmacologic method of analgesia in neonates. It has been proved to significantly reduce crying and pain response during procedures that cause mild to moderate pain, such as heel sticks and circumcision.[40,41] Although beneficial, the efficacy ends as soon as the pacifier is removed from the infant's mouth, which can in turn lead to a rebound distress response.[33]

Formula, expressed breast milk, and breastfeeding have been used for reducing infant pain. Both formula and breast milk could significantly reduce procedural pain in neonates, even though to a lesser extent compared with sucrose.[42–44] Infants receiving breastfeeding during a painful procedure have been found to demonstrate

Table 2
Nonpharmacologic pain interventions and major effects

Interventions	Major Effects: Research Evidence	Use in Painful Procedures
Sweet-tasting solutions: sucrose and glucose administration	• Decrease changes of heart rate. • Reduce crying time and facial grimacing. • Lower pain scores (PIPP and NFCS scores) • Physiologic mechanism not entirely understood; may activate endogenous opioid and nonopioid pathways through orotactile and oro-gustatory stimulation	• Effective and safe for single does given to full-term and preterm infants • Use in heel stick, intramuscular injection, venipuncture, subcutaneous injections, bladder catheterization, arterial puncture, insertion of nasogastric/orogastric tubes, eye examinations, and echocardiography • Manage short-term (5–8 min) pain and usually given 2 min before the procedure. Administer on the infant's tongue with a pacifier, syringe, or cup. • No clear recommendation of optimal dose (a 20-fold variation in the doses used) • Recommended by IASP: 24% sucrose can be given: 24–26 wk GA: 0.1 mL 27–31 wk GA: 0.25 mL 32–36 wk GA: 0.5 mL >37 wk GA: 1 mL • Concerns: potential adverse effects for repeated, multiple dose regimens in preterm infants
Skin-to-skin contact (KC)	• Decrease changes of heart rate, respiratory rate, and oxygenation saturation • Decrease crying time and facial grimacing • Improve behavioral states and sleep-wake patterns • Lower pain scores (eg, PIPP and NFCS scores) • Reduce recovery time • Decrease cortisol concentrations • Promote autonomic maturation (eg, heart rate variability) • Reduce parental stress and anxiety and increase competence • Provide multisensory stimulation; activate β-endorphin release (endogenous opioid response) and oxytocin mechanism	• Effective and safe in full-term and preterm infants • Use in heel stick, intramuscular injection, venipuncture, and subcutaneous injections, and preoperation and postoperation • Use preprocedures, during procedures, and post-procedures, 10–15 min, 30 min, 80 min, or 2–3 h • Effects last as the infant placed in the KC position and may also last after KC session

(*continued on next page*)

Table 2
(*continued*)

Interventions	Major Effects: Research Evidence	Use in Painful Procedures
NNS	• Decrease changes of heart rate, respiratory rate, and oxygenation saturation • Decrease crying time • Decrease cortisol concentrations • Lower pain scores (eg, PIPP and NFCS scores) • Mechanism of NNS on pain is unclear; may stimulate orotactile and mechanoreceptors in the mouth and regulate behavioral states	• Effective and safe in full-term and preterm infants • Use in heel stick, circumcision, intramuscular injection, venipuncture, and subcutaneous injections, and preoperation and postoperation • Administer NNS at least 3 min before the procedure • Effective when pacifier is in the infant's mouth; removal can lead to rebound distress • Best used in procedures with mild to moderate pain • Concerns: influence on initiation and sustainability of breastfeeding practice
Formula, breast milk, and breastfeeding	• Decrease changes in heart rate • Reduce crying time • Lower pain scores (eg, PIPP, NIPS, NFCS, and DAN scores)	• Safe and effective for repeated administration in full-term and preterm infants • Use in heel stick, intramuscular injection, and venipuncture • May provide similar effectiveness to oral sucrose or glucose solutions
FT	• Decrease changes in heart rate • Reduce crying time • Lower pain scores (eg, PIPP and NIPS scores) • Reduce parental stress and increase competence when parents participate in	• Safe and effective in full-term and preterm infants • Use in heel stick, endotracheal suctioning, and venipuncture • Use FT before, during, and after procedures. • Contraindication: infants with poor skin integrity (eg, extreme prematurity or epidermolysis bullosa)
Swaddling	• Decrease changes of heart rate and oxygenation saturation • Reduce crying time • Lower pain scores (eg, NIPS scores) • Shorten pain recovery time • Reduce parental stress and increase competence when parents participate in	• Safe and effective in preterm infants • Use in heel stick • Use swaddling before, during, and after procedures • Contraindication: infants with poor skin integrity (eg, extreme prematurity or epidermolysis bullosa)
Heel warming	• Decrease changes of heart rate and oxygenation saturation • Reduce crying time • Lower pain scores (eg, NIPS scores) • Shorten pain recovery time	• Safe and effective in preterm infants • Use in heel stick • Use before heel stick

Abbreviations: DAN, Douleur Aiguë du Nouveau-né score; wk GA, weeks gestational age; IASP, International Association for the Study of Pain.

a significantly lower increase in heart rate, reduced crying, and lower pain scores compared with other nonpharmacologic interventions, such as swaddling, holding, and NNS.[45]

FT is a specific way of gently holding an infant in a flexed position. It requires minimal physical adjustment and is even safe to use in mechanically ventilated neonates.[46] FT also reduces pain in neonates during painful procedures. Although beneficial, some studies indicate that it is not as efficacious as NNS.[41] Therefore, the combination of NNS and FT may be more beneficial than using FT alone.[46]

Swaddling neonates involves wrapping the neonate firmly in a blanket or other restrictive devise. Studies investigating the analgesic properties have shown that it is effective after a painful procedure, in regard to autonomic stability and recovery. Prior research indicates that swaddling may not be effective for neonates younger than 31 weeks' gestational age, although research performed by Huang and colleagues[47] has provided contradictory results.[48] Within the study, the efficacy of swaddling was seen across all age groups pertaining to oxygen saturation recovery.

Heel warming is often used during the preparatory phase prior to a heel stick. By warming a neonate's heel, there may be a reduced pain response related to the decreased need for squeezing related to increased blood flow to the area. An early study did not find a difference in infant pain perception or an improvement in analgesic effect using heel warming.[49] Conversely, a recent study found heel warming to decrease pain response during heel sticks and improve recovery time in oxygen saturation.[50] More randomized clinical trials must be performed to make a definitive conclusion as to whether or not heel warming is beneficial in providing analgesic relief.

Combining several methods of nonpharmacologic therapies via multisensory stimulation have proved most effective in providing analgesic effects.[51] The combinations of oral sucrose–FT, sucking–oral sucrose, and NNS–oral sucrose–FT have been most effective in reducing neonate crying and fussiness during routine care.[52] Use of a combination of nonpharmacologic interventions can achieve greater effectiveness of pain reduction and therefore is highly recommended in neonatal pain management.[30]

NEONATAL PAIN MANAGEMENT: PHARMACOLOGIC INTERVENTIONS

Careful consideration must be taken in administering analgesics to neonates and infants in the NICU. This is due in part to the difficulty of pain assessment, variability in individual metabolisms, neurodevelopment, and drug clearance rates, all of which can lead to adverse events and side effects.[53] Pharmacologic therapy should be administered in a stepwise approach. The type of pain that the neonate is experiencing (ie, procedural vs disease process) determines the type of analgesia best suited. The different types of pharmacologic analgesic therapies frequently used within the NICU are defined.

Opioids must be carefully administered and monitored in the neonate due to underdeveloped renal function, which results in decreased clearance due to the glomerular filtration rate. Decreased glomerular filtration rate, decreased protein binding, immature hepatic function, and the blood-brain barrier, in combination with prematurity and subsequent illness, may lead to altered opioid pharmacokinetics and possible respiratory depression in neonates.[54] Morphine is often used as the first choice of opioid analgesia in critically ill neonates, despite its known tolerance in the neonate.[55] It is broken down and metabolized within the liver, although, due to its water solubility, it has the potential to cross the neonate's blood-brain barrier leading to respiratory depression.[54,56] Due to these potentially life-threatening side effects, reduced morphine doses are necessary. There is significant evidence of opioid tolerance in neonates, which increases the need for vigilance and individualized care plans for neonates on morphine therapy. Several other opioids may be used in neonates, such as fentanyl and ketamine. Administration of opioids may be done via intermittent and/or continuous intravenous injections or oral or rectal preparations.

Nonopioid analgesics include multiple analgesic modalities, such as acetaminophen, nonsteroidal inflammatory drugs, benzodiazepines, and local and regional anesthetics. Benzodiazepines, such as midazolam and lorazepam, are often used in neonates to induce sedation and muscle relaxation. They have a limited analgesic effect, although in conjunction with other analgesic modalities, such as morphine, sedation is oftentimes improved, but due to adverse side effects, caution must be taken in administering to neonates.[53]

Regional anesthetics (ie, lidocaine) are often the analgesic of choice among neonates undergoing circumcision, as a dorsal penile block. Epidural anesthesia also may be helpful in surgical pain experienced by neonates. The use of epidural anesthesia may significantly decrease a neonate's surgical stress response as well as decrease the reduce the need for mechanical ventilation during the postoperative period.[57]

Local topical anesthetics are helpful in alleviating pain, specific to pain that is induced by breaking of the skin barrier (ie, lumbar puncture). Although this is true, topical anesthetics, such as eutectic mixture of local anesthetic, have been least effective in circumcision and heel sticks. In addition, the time of onset for topical anesthetics is often much longer than those that are regional in nature, 60 minutes to 90 minutes.[58] Eutectic mixture of local anesthetic may be helpful in producing an analgesic response during intravenous catheter insertion (peripheral and/or arterial) as well as lumbar puncture and screening for retinopathy of prematurity.[51]

BARRIERS AND PERCEPTIONS ABOUT NEONATAL PAIN

Neonatal pain management has been an enigma since 1980 when neonatal pain was first acknowledged.[59] Managing neonatal pain is a primary responsibility of neonatal nurses. Among NICU nurses, there was consensus that nurses were responsible for preventing neonate pain. They also expressed, however, that their physician counterparts did not value pain management as much as NICU nurses.[60] The commonly held paradigms about pain in the neonatal population by nurses directly influence critical decisions during neonatal care. Understanding these perceptions has only recently become a focus of nursing research and has taken on several common themes.

Neonatal nurses in the United States, the United Kingdom, and China were surveyed about their current knowledge of and beliefs about neonatal pain, assessment, intervention, and protocol as well as barriers to and strategies for improvement. It was found that nurses were generally knowledgeable about pain in neonates.[61,62] Chinese nurses held a belief that there was no difference between neonate, older child, and adult pain, indicating a knowledge gap.[63] Traditionally, Western nurses felt more comfortable using pharmacologic interventions, whereas Chinese nurses believe that nonpharmacologic interventions are efficacious for pain treatment.[62,63] Nurses in the UK reported that they were more concerned with under-medication for pain than over-medication.[62] Fewer than half of the Chinese nurses knew of the pain management protocols in their unit and a majority of American, UK, and Chinese nurses believed that the protocols were unclear and not based on the evidence of neonatal pain research.[61–63] This leads to the conclusion that there is an important gap in the way in which nurses evaluate and manage neonatal pain.

Narrative data collected from American, UK, and Chinese nurses revealed the barriers to pain management were lack of time, knowledge, and trust in the tools used, the latter two likely contributing to reported fear and reluctance to change current practice.[62,63] It was suggested that education and utilization of research along with improved communication would improve pain management.

SUMMARY

Neonatal infants, especially preterm infants, are most likely to experience a great number of repeated and prolonged painful events in the NICU that can lead to deleterious consequences, including neurodevelopmental impairment, as a result. Appropriate steps have been taken to ensure a paradigm shift regarding neonatal pain and its processing and management. A deeper understanding of the pain sensory mechanism and its ramifications is necessary for a more accommodating neonatal health care practice. Nonpharmacologic interventions, especially those incorporating parental involvement (eg, KC) are highly recommended. To discover new and creative approaches to address the challenge of infant pain is a primary nursing focus. According to the clinical, ethical,[64] and policy statements,[4,65,66] developing optimal assessment and treatment techniques to reduce neonatal pain is an important topic and challenge for neonatal caregivers. Even though there are gaps in knowledge, practice, attitudes, and policy regarding infant pain, health care providers should implement pain management programs to assess, prevent, and relieve pain in neonates using nonpharmacologic and pharmacologic strategies.

REFERENCES

1. Anand KJ, Hickey PR. Pain and its effects in the human neonate and fetus. N Engl J Med 1987;317(21):1321–9.
2. Fitzgerald M, Beggs S. The neurobiology of pain: developmental aspects. Neuroscientist 2001;7(3):246–57.
3. Grunau RE, Holsti L, Haley D, et al. Neonatal procedural pain exposure predicts lower cortisol and behavioral reactivity in preterm infants in the NICU. Pain 2005; 113(3):293–300.
4. Committee On F, Newborn, Section On A, et al. Prevention and management of procedural pain in the neonate: an update. Pediatrics 2016;137(2):e20154271.
5. Goksan S, Hartley C, Emery F, et al. fMRI reveals neural activity overlap between adult and infant pain. Elife 2015;4.
6. Cong X, Wu J, Vittner D, et al. The impact of cumulative pain/stress on neurobehavioral development of preterm infants in the NICU. Early Hum Dev 2017;108: 9–16.
7. Lippmann M, Nelson RJ, Emmanouilides GC, et al. Ligation of patent ductus arteriosus in premature infants. Br J Anaesth 1976;48(4):365–9.
8. Holsti L, Grunau RE, Shany E. Assessing pain in preterm infants in the neonatal intensive care unit: moving to a 'brain-oriented' approach. Pain Manag 2011;1(2): 171–9.
9. In: Osterweis M, Kleinman A, Mechanic D, editors. Pain and disability: clinical, behavioral, and public policy perspectives. Washington, DC: National Academies Press (US); 1987. Available from: https://www.ncbi.nlm.nih.gov/books/NBK219254/ doi: 10.17226/991.
10. Brown AG. The dorsal horn of the spinal cord. Q J Exp Physiol 1982;67(2): 193–212.

11. Ab Aziz CB, Ahmad AH. The role of the thalamus in modulating pain. Malays J Med Sci 2006;13(2):11–8.
12. Hatfield LA. Neonatal pain: what's age got to do with it? Surg Neurol Int 2014; 5(Suppl 13):S479–89.
13. Kostovic I, Rakic P. Developmental history of the transient subplate zone in the visual and somatosensory cortex of the macaque monkey and human brain. J Comp Neurol 1990;297(3):441–70.
14. Hasegawa M, Houdou S, Mito T, et al. Development of myelination in the human fetal and infant cerebrum: a myelin basic protein immunohistochemical study. Brain Dev 1992;14(1):1–6.
15. Dubin AE, Patapoutian A. Nociceptors: the sensors of the pain pathway. J Clin Invest 2010;120(11):3760–72.
16. Fitzgerald M, Walker SM. Infant pain management: a developmental neurobiological approach. Nat Clin Pract Neurol 2009;5(1):35–50.
17. Slater R, Fabrizi L, Worley A, et al. Premature infants display increased noxious-evoked neuronal activity in the brain compared to healthy age-matched term-born infants. Neuroimage 2010;52(2):583–9.
18. Cong X, McGrath JM, Cusson RM, et al. Pain assessment and measurement in neonates: an updated review. Adv Neonatal Care 2013;13(6):379–95.
19. Ranger M, Grunau RE. Early repetitive pain in preterm infants in relation to the developing brain. Pain Manag 2014;4(1):57–67.
20. Xu W, Walsh S, Cong XS. Development of accumulated pain/stressor scale (APSS) in NICUs: a national survey. Pain Manag Nurs 2016;17(6):354–62.
21. Grunau RE, Craig KD. Pain expression in neonates: facial action and cry. Pain 1987;28(3):395–410.
22. Hummel P, Puchalski M, Creech SD, et al. Clinical reliability and validity of the N-PASS: neonatal pain, agitation and sedation scale with prolonged pain. J Perinatol 2008;28(1):55–60.
23. van Dijk M, Roofthooft DW, Anand KJ, et al. Taking up the challenge of measuring prolonged pain in (premature) neonates: the COMFORTneo scale seems promising. Clin J Pain 2009;25(7):607–16.
24. Lawrence J, Alcock D, McGrath P, et al. The development of a tool to assess neonatal pain. Neonatal Netw 1993;12(6):59–66.
25. Crellin DJ, Harrison D, Santamaria N, et al. Systematic review of the Face, Legs, Activity, Cry and Consolability scale for assessing pain in infants and children: is it reliable, valid, and feasible for use? Pain 2015;156(11):2132–51.
26. Stevens BJ, Gibbins S, Yamada J, et al. The premature infant pain profile-revised (PIPP-R): initial validation and feasibility. Clin J Pain 2014;30(3):238–43.
27. Cong X, Cusson RM, Walsh S, et al. Effects of skin-to-skin contact on autonomic pain responses in preterm infants. J Pain 2012;13(7):636–45.
28. Tristao RM, Garcia NV, de Jesus JA, et al. COMFORT behaviour scale and skin conductance activity: what are they really measuring? Acta Paediatr 2013; 102(9):e402–6.
29. Hartley C, Slater R. Neurophysiological measures of nociceptive brain activity in the newborn infant–the next steps. Acta Paediatr 2014;103(3):238–42.
30. IASP IAftSoP. Acute pain management in newborn infants. Pain Clinical Updates. 2011. Available at: http://www.iasp-pain.org/AM/AMTemplate.cfm?Section=IASP_Press_Books2&CONTENTID=15068&SECTION=IASP_Press_Books2&TEMPLATE=/CM/ContentDisplay.cfm. Accessed December 13, 2017.

31. Gao H, Gao H, Xu G, et al. Efficacy and safety of repeated oral sucrose for repeated procedural pain in neonates: a systematic review. Int J Nurs Stud 2016;62:118–25.
32. Stevens B, Yamada J, Ohlsson A, et al. Sucrose for analgesia in newborn infants undergoing painful procedures. Cochrane Database Syst Rev 2016;(7):CD001069.
33. Gibbins S, Stevens B. Mechanisms of sucrose and non-nutritive sucking in procedural pain management in infants. Pain Res Manag 2001;6(1):21–8.
34. Cong X, Ludington-Hoe SM, Walsh S. Randomized crossover trial of kangaroo care to reduce biobehavioral pain responses in preterm infants: a pilot study. Biol Res Nurs 2011;13(2):204–16.
35. Boundy EO, Dastjerdi R, Spiegelman D, et al. Kangaroo mother care and neonatal outcomes: a meta-analysis. Pediatrics 2016;137(1):1–16.
36. Johnston CC, Filion F, Campbell-Yeo M, et al. Kangaroo mother care diminishes pain from heel lance in very preterm neonates: a crossover trial. BMC Pediatr 2008;8:13.
37. Cong X, Ludington-Hoe SM, McCain G, et al. Kangaroo Care modifies preterm infant heart rate variability in response to heel stick pain: pilot study. Early Hum Dev 2009;85(9):561–7.
38. Ludington-Hoe S, Hosseini R, Torowicz DL. Skin-to-skin contact (Kangaroo Care) analgesia for preterm infant heel stick. AACN Clin Issues 2005;16(3):373–87.
39. Vittner D, McGrath J, Robinson J, et al. Increase in oxytocin from skin-to-skin contact enhances development of parent-infant relationship. Biol Res Nurs 2018;20(1):54–62.
40. Golianu B, Krane E, Seybold J, et al. Non-pharmacological techniques for pain management in neonates. Semin Perinatol 2007;31(5):318–22.
41. Liaw JJ, Yang L, Katherine Wang KW, et al. Non-nutritive sucking and facilitated tucking relieve preterm infant pain during heel-stick procedures: a prospective, randomised controlled crossover trial. Int J Nurs Stud 2012;49(3):300–9.
42. Collados-Gomez L, Ferrera-Camacho P, Fernandez-Serrano E, et al. Randomised crossover trial showed that using breast milk or sucrose provided the same analgesic effect in preterm infants of at least 28 weeks. Acta Paediatr 2018;107(3):436–41.
43. Blass EM. Milk-induced hypoalgesia in human newborns. Pediatrics 1997;99(6):825–9.
44. Ou-Yang MC, Chen IL, Chen CC, et al. Expressed breast milk for procedural pain in preterm neonates: a randomized, double-blind, placebo-controlled trial. Acta Paediatr 2013;102(1):15–21.
45. Shah PS, Herbozo C, Aliwalas LL, et al. Breastfeeding or breast milk for procedural pain in neonates. Cochrane Database Syst Rev 2012;(12):CD004950.
46. Hartley KA, Miller CS, Gephart SM. Facilitated tucking to reduce pain in neonates: evidence for best practice. Adv Neonatal Care 2015;15(3):201–8.
47. Huang CM, Tung WS, Kuo LL, et al. Comparison of pain responses of premature infants to the heelstick between containment and swaddling. J Nurs Res 2004;12(1):31–40.
48. Cignacco E, Hamers JP, Stoffel L, et al. The efficacy of non-pharmacological interventions in the management of procedural pain in preterm and term neonates. A systematic literature review. Eur J Pain 2007;11(2):139–52.
49. Barker DP, Willetts B, Cappendijk VC, et al. Capillary blood sampling: should the heel be warmed? Arch Dis Child Fetal Neonatal Ed 1996;74(2):F139–40.

50. Shu SH, Lee YL, Hayter M, et al. Efficacy of swaddling and heel warming on pain response to heel stick in neonates: a randomised control trial. J Clin Nurs 2014; 23(21–22):3107–14.
51. Krishnan L. Pain relief in neonates. J Neonatal Surg 2013;2(2):19.
52. Liaw JJ, Yang L, Lee CM, et al. Effects of combined use of non-nutritive sucking, oral sucrose, and facilitated tucking on infant behavioural states across heel-stick procedures: a prospective, randomised controlled trial. Int J Nurs Stud 2013; 50(7):883–94.
53. Hall RW, Shbarou RM. Drugs of choice for sedation and analgesia in the neonatal ICU. Clin Perinatol 2009;36(2):215–26, vii.
54. Bhalla T, Shepherd E, Tobias JD. Neonatal pain management. Saudi J Anaesth 2014;8(Suppl 1):S89–97.
55. Hall RW. Anesthesia and analgesia in the NICU. Clin Perinatol 2012;39(1):239–54.
56. Haidon JL, Cunliffe M. Analgesia for neonates. Continuing Education in Anaesthesia Critical Care and Pain 2010;10(4):123–7.
57. Lönnqvist PA. Regional anesthesia and analgesia in the neonate. Best Pract Res Clin Anaesthesiol 2010;24(3):309–21.
58. Anand K, Johnston C, Oberlander T, et al. Analgesia and local anesthesia during invasive procedures in the neonate. Clin Ther 2005;27(6):844–76.
59. Anand K, Hall W. Controversies in neonatal pain: an introduction. Semin Perinatol 2007;31(5):273–4.
60. Byrd PJ, Gonzales I, Parsons V. Exploring barriers to pain management in newborn intensive care units: a pilot survey of NICU nurses. Adv Neonatal Care 2009;9(6):299–306.
61. Cong X, Delaney C, Vazquez V. Neonatal nurses' perceptions of pain assessment and management in NICUs: a national survey. Adv Neonatal Care 2013;13(5): 353–60.
62. Akuma AO, Jordan S. Pain management in neonates: a survey of nurses and doctors. J Adv Nurs 2012;68(6):1288–301.
63. Cong X, McGrath JM, Delaney C, et al. Neonatal nurses' perceptions of pain management: survey of the United States and China. Pain Manag Nurs 2014; 15(4):834–44.
64. Franck LS. A pain in the act: musings on the meaning for critical care nurses of the pain management standards of the joint commission on accreditation of healthcare organizations. Crit Care Nurse 2001;21(3):8, 10, 12 passim.
65. Prevention and Management of Procedural Pain in the Neonate: An Update. COMMITTEE ON FETUS AND NEWBORN and SECTION ON ANESTHESIOLOGY AND PAIN MEDICINE Pediatrics Feb 2016;137(2):e20154271; https://doi.org/10.1542/peds.2015-4271.
66. Baker DW. Statement on pain management: understanding how joint commission standards address pain. Jt Comm Perspect 2016;36(6):10–2.
67. Merkel SI, Vopel-Lewis T, Shayevitz JR, et al. The FLACC: a behavioral scale for scoring postoperative pain in young children. Pediatr Nurs 1997;23(3):293–7.
68. Stevens B, Johnston C, Petryshen P, et al. Premature Infant Pain Profile: development and initial validation. Clin J Pain 1996;12(1):13–22.

Neuroprotective Care of Extremely Preterm Infants in the First 72 Hours After Birth

Leslie Altimier, DNP, RN, MSN, NE-BC[a,b,*],
Raylene Phillips, MD, MA, IBCLC[c,d]

KEYWORDS

- Neuroprotection • Neonatal • Integrative • Developmental care • Core measures
- Small baby programs

KEY POINTS

- Neuro-supportive and neuroprotective family-centered developmental care and standardized care practices for extremely preterm infants have been shown to improve outcomes.
- Neuroprotective skin-to-skin contact with mother is the developmentally expected environment for all mammals and is especially important for supporting physiological stability and optimal neurodevelopment in preterm infants.
- Neuroprotective interventions must include a focus on the interpersonal experiences and emotional connections of infants and their families in the NICU.
- For optimal neurodevelopmental outcomes, neonatal intensive care unit staff should be experts in providing both clinical and neuroprotective support to babies and psychosocial support to parents and families.

INTRODUCTION

Birth at extremely low gestational ages presents a significant threat to an infant's survival, health, development, and future well-being. Although comprising just 1% to 2% of all births, extremely preterm (EP) infants (delivered at 22–28 weeks' gestation) pose the greatest challenge to neonatal medicine, health care, education, and social services in providing ongoing support for survivors who often have significant ongoing needs. A population-based study determined that 28% of all EP infants died within

Disclosure: The authors have nothing to disclose.
[a] Northeastern University, School of Nursing in the Bouvé College of Health Sciences, 360 Huntington Avenue, Boston, MA 02115, USA; [b] Philips HealthTech, Cambridge, MA, USA; [c] Loma Linda University School of Medicine, Department of Pediatrics, Division of Neonatology, Loma Linda University Children's Hospital, 11175 Campus Street, CP 11121 Loma Linda, CA 92354, USA; [d] Loma Linda University Medical Center-Murrieta, 28062 Baxter Road, Murrieta, CA 92563, USA
* Corresponding author. 35 Warren Street, Newburyport, MA 01950.
E-mail address: LAltimier@gmail.com

Crit Care Nurs Clin N Am 30 (2018) 563–583
https://doi.org/10.1016/j.cnc.2018.07.010

the first year of life. Among infants born at 22, 23, and 24 weeks, survival to 1 year of age was 6%, 27%, and 60%, respectively, and increased for each 1-week increase in gestational age from 78% at 25 weeks to 94% at 28 weeks.[1] Although survival rates for extremely low birthweight (ELBW) premature infants have improved, there has only been a modest improvement in the proportion of surviving infants without neurologic impairment, no change in the proportion with severe disability, and an overall increase in the total number of children with neuro-disability.[2]

Despite the continually evolving and less invasive strategies used to care for premature infants in the neonatal intensive care unit (NICU), the prevalence of major neonatal morbidities common to this gestational age group, chronic lung disease (CLD) or bronchopulmonary dysplasia (BPD), periventricular leukomalacia (PVL), intraventricular hemorrhage (IVH), cerebral palsy (CP), necrotizing enterocolitis (NEC), retinopathy of prematurity (ROP), severe visual and hearing impairment, and sepsis, is essentially unchanged.[3] Increasing numbers of premature infants are being discharged from the hospital and sent home on oxygen with apnea monitors, gastrostomy or nasogastric tubes, and high-calorie formulas. Infants discharged from a NICU after a lengthy hospitalization have much higher rates of rehospitalizations during their first year of life than their full-term peers.[4]

As we strive to improve morbidity and mortality rates, we are challenged to enhance current neuroprotective strategies for prematurely born infants that include a focus on the interpersonal experiences and emotional connections of the infant and their family in the NICU. Infants born prematurely have demonstrated markedly improved outcomes when the stress of environmental overstimulation is reduced and family bonds are supported, which can be accomplished by providing neuro-supportive care and incorporating neuroprotective interventions (NPIs) into the care of high-risk neonates.[5]

The concept of neuroprotection is not new to the medical field; however, the idea that NPIs provided by multidisciplinary NICU staff (medical, nursing, and therapy) may promote normal development of the premature infant's brain has been more difficult to prove.[6–8] There are several antenatal NPIs that can be implemented at the onset of premature labor; however, once delivered, the preterm brain must continue critical neurologic growth and maturation in the often-times harsh extrauterine NICU environment.

Neurodevelopment of the Fetal Brain

Development of the central nervous system is divided into 6 overlapping stages: neurulation, prosencephalic development, neuronal proliferation, neuronal migration, organization, and myelination. Organization allows the nervous system to act as an integrated whole and is where the development of synaptic connections (wiring of the brain) as well as cell death and selective elimination of excess neuronal processes is occurring. The peak period for organization starts around the fifth month of gestation, which is when extremely prematurely born infants are now growing in the NICU environment.[5,9]

The architecture of connections in the brain are made with dendritic growth, synaptic networks, apoptosis, myelination, and pruning. Research shows that outside stimulation from the environment can induce changes in the pattern of brain development designed to occur in the last trimester of pregnancy and in early life, altering the development and impacting the quality of these connections.

MRI's performed on the brains of infants born 10 weeks prematurely showed 30% less gray matter (the brain's thinking cells) and 40% less white matter (connections in the brain).[10] Hebbian Associative Learning was derived by Donald Hebb in 1949 and includes what is now known as Hebb's law. Although Hebb's law states that "neurons that fire together, wire together," it implies that "neurons that don't, won't," or that "neurons that fire apart, wire apart."[11] This idea means that repeated experiences (positive or negative) reinforce particular patterns of synaptic connections (wiring) and a lack of appropriate experiences diminishes the firing of neurons, impacting the ability to hard wire synapses, thus, altering the developing brain. NPIs support the developing brain and facilitate healing of the brain after a neuron injury by decreasing neuronal death and by promoting the development of new connections and pathways for functionality.[12]

Neuro-supportive Care

Although *neuroprotective* care helps to protect the preterm brain from the relatively harsh, extrauterine environment of the NICU, *neuro-supportive* care provides a foundation on which neuroprotection can occur. Dr Nils Bergman[13] and others have made a strong case for the neuro-supportive nature of skin-to-skin contact (SSC) between newborn infants and their parents. "The optimal environment for any newborn, but particularly for the premature infant, is skin-to-skin contact with mother (or father), also known as kangaroo care."[13] For all primates, the mother's womb is the normal environment where development begins and the mother's body is the normal environment where development continues after birth. In SSC, the newborn receives salient and expected sensory inputs that lead to physiologic regulation and a secure attachment, processes that are both mediated by the limbic system and essential for normal development. Dr Bergman[13] asserts that SSC is, therefore, not a care practice but is a place where all neuroprotective care practices would ideally be done. Skin-to-skin care is not an intervention but is our biological default.

In most NICU cultures, the incubator is seen as the normal environment for premature infants and maternal-infant separation is seen as unavoidable and of little consequence. However, separation from the mother is highly abnormal to all newborns, no matter how prematurely they are born, and is known to alter physiologic stability, epigenes, DNA, and the developing brain.[13,14] Separated neonates experience a state of anxious arousal when separated from maternal presence, which is their biologically expected place of warmth, nutrition, and safety. If SSC with the mother or father is not promptly reestablished, the neonate's autonomic nervous system triggers a sequence of responses leading to freeze and dissociation, a terror state in which the brain tunes out. These 3 responses are often mistaken for sleep but can be distinguished from sleep both clinically and electronically.[15] Much attention has been given to toxic stress, which is defined as stress experienced in the absence of the buffering presence of adult support. The goal of NICU care should be to ensure there is never an "absence of the buffering presence of adult support" and that support should come from the primary attachment figures for the neonate whenever possible.

Because of the well-document high level of stress to the newborn caused by separation from the mother, Dr Bergman[16] recommends zero separation. There are situations whereby a mother and infant must be separated, particularly if the mother is ill or unable to be present; however, zero separation is the biological default and should be the goal. Bergman and colleagues[17] have provided convincing evidence in 2 randomized controlled trials that healthy preterm infants are more physiologically stable in SSC with their mothers during the first 6 hours after birth than separated from their mothers while inside an incubator.[18] There is no standard recommendation or definition for SSC eligibility. Infants may be labeled ineligible for technical reasons, for staff competency or shift change reasons, and a host of other issues; however, there is no real medical or scientific contraindication, because separation is the core cause of so many adverse outcomes. There are some units that limit SSC in the first 24 to 72 hours after birth because of concerns about altering cerebral blood flow and increasing the risk of IVH from head movement and neck position in extremely premature infants; however, this concern is not substantiated by evidence. Liao and colleagues[19] found head position change did not alter cerebral oxygenation and found no significant effect of head position or head tilting on the incidence of IVH. We need to move beyond seeing SSC as an intervention to be done after an infant has been stabilized to seeing SSC as the place where the infant is most likely to become and remain stable.

Neurodevelopmental Risks of Prematurity

Following delivery, physiologic instability and systemic inflammation (exacerbated by separation from mother) predispose the preterm brain to IVH and white matter damage.[20] Infants born early are susceptible to alterations in brain development not only because of the disruption of genetically programmed patterns of brain genesis, but also because of experiences, such as neurologic insults, including IVH and PVL; biological influences, such as infection, BPD, and ROP; and environmental influences, such as altered auditory and visual stimuli, along with physical separation from their parents. Despite many advances in obstetric and neonatal care that have improved neurobehavioral outcomes for preterm children over the past few decades,[12] the rates of impairments remain too high; early NPIs are needed during the neonatal intensive care period and especially during the first 72 hours after birth to optimize outcomes.[21–24]

Neuro-supportive care along with medically driven NPIs can assist in preventing and minimizing negative outcomes. The following diseases and associated NPIs are discussed: IVH, apnea of prematurity (AOP), patent ductus arteriosus (PDA), late-onset sepsis (LOS), ROP, NEC, and low Mental Developmental Index (MDI) scores.

IVH is a significant cause of moderate-severe brain injury in preterm infants, with most occurring within the first 72 hours after birth. Both deferred or delayed cord clamping and cord milking are postnatal NPIs that have led to a reduction in mortality and multisystem morbidity in preterm infants, including anemia and all grades of IVH.[25–27]

In some studies, indomethacin prophylaxis has been shown to significantly reduce the incidence of severe IVH and leads to a borderline significant reduction in ventriculomegaly, PVL, or other white matter echo abnormalities but did not change survival rates or long-term developmental outcomes; practice remains varied.[28–30]

AOP affects almost all infants born at less than 28 weeks' gestation or with a birth weight less than 1000 g. When untreated, AOP may be associated with negative outcomes; therefore, effective treatment of AOP is an important part of optimizing care of preterm infants.[31,32] In a randomized controlled trial, prophylactic treatment of AOP with caffeine in the first 10 days was found to decrease the incidence of CP and cognitive impairment at 18 to 21 months in low-birth-weight at-risk infants.[33] Studies suggest that starting caffeine early, in the first 1 to 3 days of life, is beneficial with reductions in death, BPD, and PDA.[34,35]

Closure of the PDA is delayed in up to 80% of infants born at less than 25 weeks' gestational age and as many as 70% of infants born at less than 28 weeks' gestational age.[36] PDA can be associated with IVH and abnormalities of cerebral perfusion.[36] Currently, management of PDA remains controversial because many resolve without intervention and many that persist do not become clinically significant.[37,38] It has been hypothesized that neurologic detriment actually occurs before the PDA becomes clinically significant.[39]

Late Onset Sepsis, Necrotizing Enterocolitis, and poor nutritional status are associated with adverse neurodevelopmental outcomes in preterm infants.[40–42] Approximately 21% to 36% of very-low-birthweight preterm infants have LOS.[40,41,43] Neurodevelopmental impairment is increased following clinical infection as well as culture-positive sepsis and meningitis when compared with infants without suspected sepsis.[44] Standardized care bundles for central lines decrease infections by up to 67%.[45] Implementation of such a bundle resulted in improved cognitive outcome at 2 years of age in one report.[46] Antimicrobial stewardship, limited postnatal steroid use, early enteral feeding with breast milk, and meticulous hand hygiene are also important and cost-effective strategies for reducing the burden of LOS.[45] Receiving human milk not only protects against LOS, NEC, and death but it also has been linked to many other improved outcomes. One study demonstrated that infants receiving feedings of human milk achieved full enteral nutrition sooner, required shorter duration of central venous lines, had fewer episodes of pneumonia, had less incidence of NEC, and had less PVL than infants fed exclusively preterm formula.[47] In one Swedish study, the most influential risk factor for LOS was the number of days without establishment of full enteral feeds with human milk. Growing evidence supports the role of probiotics in reducing the risk of NEC, time to achieve full enteral feeding, and LOS in preterm infants.[48]

Retinopathy of prematurity (ROP) is a multifactorial vasoproliferative disorder of eye development related to prematurity that affects up to 40–80% of preterm neonates with frequency inversely correlated to birth weight and gestational age.[49] ROP incidence is increasing worldwide as a consequence of the higher survival rates of preterm neonates.[50] ROP is still a leading cause of blindness in babies born prematurity secondary to retinal detachment.[51] Human milk feeding is indicated for all premature infants as it provides superior nutritional and immunological benefits compared to formula made from bovine milk.[52] Exclusive human milk feeding has been shown to reduce the incidence and severity of ROP in VLBW infants in the NICU.[53–55] Human milk in even small quantities (< 20% of an ELBW infant's diet) has been shown to be protective against ROP, whereas greater than 60% human milk virtually eliminated severe ROP in a study by Hylander and colleagues.[56] Additionally, strategies to maintain oxygen saturations within predetermined ranges have also been shown to reduce the incidence and severity of ROP.[57,58]

Necrotizing enterocolitis (NEC) is a devastating disease characterized by damage to intestinal mucosa, which is hypothesized to involve ischemia and/or an exaggerated inflammatory response to pathogenic bacteria. The vast majority of those affected by NEC are premature infants and despite significant focus over the past decades, the pathophysiology remains incompletely understood. NEC continues to be a significant cause of mortality among EP infants,[59] and surviving NEC is associated with brain injury and poor neurodevelopmental outcomes.[60,61] NEC requiring surgery is associated with worse outcomes than NEC treated with antibiotics and withholding feeds,[53–55, 60,62–64] and the duration of NEC is proportional to neurodisability.[60] It is postulated that the systemic inflammatory response associated with NEC leads to brain injury; thus, interventions to reduce NEC rates can be deemed neuroprotective.[60] Such efforts have included the use of probiotics,[65] lactoferrin,[66] promotion of human milk feedings,[67] avoidance of bovine products,[67,68] and preventing infection, all of which are likely to be beneficial.[69] Meinzen-Derr and colleagues[70] (2009) found that the proportion of infants who survived free of NEC was correlated with the total amount of human milk they received in the first 14 days of life. Human milk provides a clear protective effect against NEC, with an approximate 4–6% reduction in incidence.[55] Sisk (2007) found that infants receiving enteral feedings containing at least 50% human milk in the first 14 days of life was associated with a sixfold decrease in the odds of NEC.[67]

Neurodevelopmental outcomes and MDI scores are improved when babies are given consistent individualized developmental care from birth.[71] Preterm infants fed with predominantly human milk were found to have increased deep nuclear gray matter volume at term corrected age,[71] improved developmental scores at 18 months,[72] and higher IQ and academic achievement at 7 years.[73] The benefits of early nutrition with human milk, including fortification, outweigh the risks of introducing enteral feeds to very preterm infants.[74] Vohr studied the effects of feeding human milk to preterm infants and found that each additional 10 mL/kg/d of human milk over the NICU stay resulted in an increase of 0.5 points in MDI, 0.6 points in the psychomotor developmental index, 0.8 points in the behavior rating scale score and a decrease of 6% in risk of rehospitalization at 18 months of age.[72] These results were found to persist at 30 months with an increase in MDI by 0.8 points for every 10-mL increase in human milk volume per kilogram per day.[74] Isaacs and colleagues[75] found the beneficial effects of a human milk diet for preterm infants was still seen in their adolescence. The percentage of expressed breast milk ingested was correlated with increased verbal IQ and white matter volume in both boys and girls and increased total brain volume in boys only. Sammallahti and colleagues[76] also confirmed that human milk intake predicted better neurocognitive abilities in adulthood as well as a higher adult IQ. Schanler and colleagues demonstrated that premature infants receiving any human milk in the NICU had higher mental and motor developmental scores as well as higher behavior rating scores.[77]

Care of Small Babies: Small Baby Programs

Babies born at 27 weeks' gestation or earlier are often called micropreemies. Beginning at the moment of birth, these very tiny babies have complex needs and developmental challenges.

To address the unique needs of these fragile babies, a new conceptual model for providing care has evolved: small baby programs (SBPs) with small baby units. The health care needs of 500-g infants are very different from those of 1500-g infants or those of average-size term infants. Because these unique differences bring unique challenges, SBPs are opening within NICUs across the country with the intent of providing focused care to micropreemies and their families. There is no clear gestational age cutoff for SBPs; however, most SBPs have established a gestational age of 27 or 28 weeks or less and some have included an upper birth weight limit of 1000 or 1250 g.

Many NICUs have cared for tiny preterm babies for decades using established care bundles, guidelines, policies, and procedures and have been considered experts in the delivery of small baby care. Although providing expert care for small babies is not new, the development of SBPs and the creation of small baby units acknowledge that this super-sub-specialty population benefits from specialized care. At the heart of this care is the prioritization of consistent and standardized care, which is accomplished through the implementation of evidence-based protocols and guidelines provided by a dedicated SBP specialty care team whose multidisciplinary members have been educated and trained in SBP practices and who have the proficiency and skill needed to handle fragile ELBW infants. In addition to knowledge of the standardized care practices, staff caring for ELBW infants should receive education about the intricacies of doing (or supporting) procedures on such tiny infants (i.e. intubations), establishing and managing non-invasive ventilation, and routine cares while maintaining a neuroprotective, healing environment at all times. Around the world, significant variations in outcomes among NICUs have been reported.[78] Practice variation among providers at the same institution are common.[78–82] Collaborative quality improvement (QI) and interdisciplinary team-based care have been shown to significantly improve outcomes.[38–51,60–76,78–85] These results likely reflect the benefits of standardized practices.[86,87] Improved outcomes and decreased length of hospitalization have been achieved through the utilization of standardized ELBW guidelines for infants during just the first 7 days of life.[88] Some SBPs have extended this concept through the entire hospitalization and have shown significant improvement in survival and clinical outcomes as well as reduced resource utilization by the implementation of standardized small baby practices and guidelines.[89] One such unit experienced a decrease in hospital-acquired infections, a decrease in growth restriction, a reduction in the incidence of CLD, an improvement in resource utilization via decreased blood tests and radiographs, as well as an improvement in staff perceptions of team support and quality of care.[89]

Small baby guidelines (SBGs) must be regularly updated with the most current best practices available. Sharek and colleagues,[90] found that the establishment of guidelines led to accelerated implementation of clinical practices that would not likely occur otherwise. Although it is interesting to speculate on what aspects of the SBG resulted in the improvements in outcomes noted, data clearly demonstrate that it is the implementation of standard guidelines for care resulting in a uniformed approach to these patients that lead to improved patient outcomes. This suggests that it is perhaps not so much what exactly the guidelines dictate (ie, what medications, fluids), but rather the standardized approach to patient care that it is the embraced by the entire health care team that leads to a change in culture and the observed benefits in patient outcomes.[88]

Multiple models have been introduced to support NICU staff in improving care of very preterm infants. Transformational change practices and neuroprotective education (Wee Care Program, Philips HealthTech, Andover, MA) have demonstrated long-standing positive results from specialized training of NICU staff in the neuroprotective family-centered developmental care of preterm infants and their families.[91–95] Positive results from staff trained in the NIDCAP approach to family-centered development care have been demonstrated for years.[71,96]

In addition to improving neonatal clinical outcomes, a primary goal of an SBP is to improve family satisfaction by providing continuity of care through dedicated SBU staff as well as by providing a unique environment for families to network with other families experiencing similar complications, lengths of hospitalization, and outcomes. It is well documented that parents of NICU babies have significantly higher rates of postpartum depression (PPD), posttraumatic stress disorder (PTSD) and anxiety disorders.[97] The psychosocial needs of parents who are enduring the unexpected and extreme stress of having a hospitalized preterm or sick newborn has been long neglected and most NICU staff (medical, nursing, and therapy) have not been trained to recognize the psychosocial needs of NICU parents. While much support can readily be given by compassionate, caring, trained NICU staff, some parents will require referral to mental health professionals. Since neurodevelopment outcomes of NICU babies are directly linked to secure attachments with their parents, supporting NICU parents in developing bonds of attachment with their babies can be considered to be neuroprotective care.

Because parental wellbeing is linked to infant wellbeing, education and training should be provided to NICU staff about how to best support NICU parents and families who are enduring the crisis of having a baby in the NICU. Interdisciplinary recommendations as well as online education and resources for providing psychosocial support to NICU parents have been recently developed by the National Perinatal Association to be used by NICU staff and families.[98–100] NICU staff will also need education and training about any new guidelines and caregiving techniques for this special population.

Neuroprotective Care

The Neonatal Integrative Developmental Care (NIDC) model (Philips HealthTech, Cambridge, MA) can be used as a framework to guide the implementation of neuroprotective care for premature infants in the first 72 hours of life. The NIDC model uses NPIs as strategies to support optimal synaptic neural connections; promote normal neurologic, physical, and emotional development; and prevent disabilities. Seven core measures for neuroprotective family-centered developmental care of premature infants are depicted on petals of a lotus as the healing environment, partnering with families, positioning and handling, safeguarding sleep, minimizing stress and pain, protecting skin, and optimizing nutrition (**Fig. 1**). The overlapping petals of the model demonstrate the integrative nature of developmental care.[6] The mother/child dyad is in the center of the lotus surrounded closely by symbols representing various aspects of the healing environment, highlighting the physical, extrauterine environment in which the infant now lives, the significance of the developing infant's sensory system, and the influence people (patient, family, and staff) have on the infant-family unit. SSC is considered the foundation for care of infants in the NICU and is the ideal environment for care to be provided. Each of the 7 distinct core measures identified in the NIDC model provides clinical guidance for NICU staff.[5–7] Appendix 1 provides a look at the NIDC model with a list of quick tips on how to implement the 7 core measures for neuroprotective family centered developmental care.

Every baby, regardless of gestational age, deserves neuroprotective care throughout their hospitalization because of the rapid brain growth and neurologic development occurring during the early neonatal period. The earlier in gestation a baby is born, the more vulnerable is its fragile brain and the more critical it is to provide effective and consistent neuroprotective care from the moment of birth and throughout their in order to protect and support optimal brain development. As the age of viability continues to decrease (for some, 22 weeks is the new 24 weeks), we must continue making strides toward improving morbidity and mortality rates, while further enhancing NPIs for these EP infants. SBPs can help to achieve this goal with

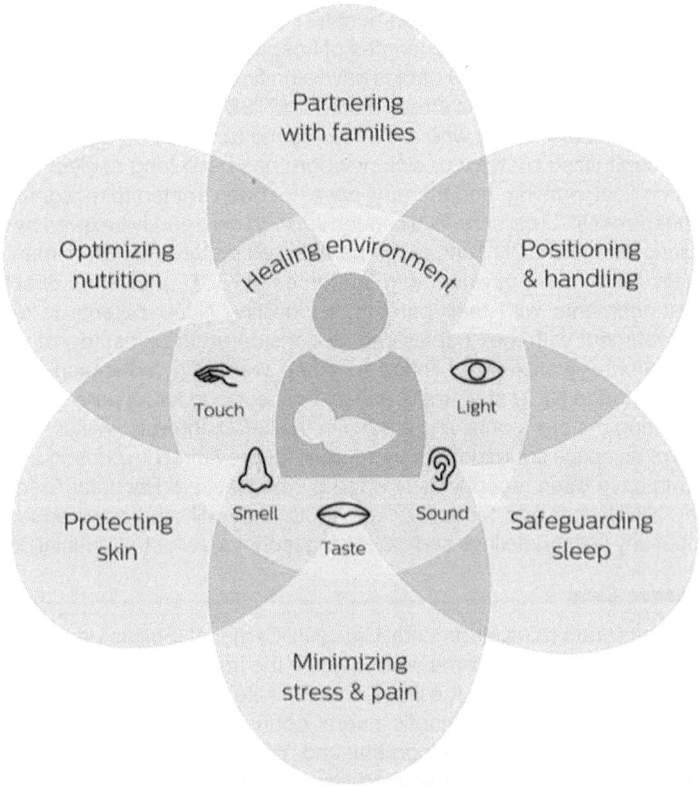

Fig. 1. NIDC model. (*Courtesy of* Koninklijke Philips N.V., Cambridge, MA; with permission.)

a dedicated highly trained staff providing consistent care through the implementation of standardized and detailed care bundles. An example of this standardized approach to care is shown in Appendix 2, which provides an example of a nursing checklist for the care of EP infants during the first 3 days after birth.

No matter how vigilantly we care for babies in the NICU, it is important to recognize that every interaction with a preterm infant affects brain development and contributes to the overall developmental outcome of the infant. There is ample evidence that neuroprotective family centered developmental care in the NICU results in improved neonatal and neurodevelopmental outcomes, increased family satisfaction, and even enhanced employee satisfaction once a culture of change has been established.[71,101–104] Both the risk of initial brain injury and subsequent neurodevelopmental problems can be reduced by optimizing currently approved and recommended best practices.[5–7,105] By consistently applying the principles and practices we know to be beneficial for extremely premature infants, we can improve the NICU experience for babies, families, and staff and make a significant difference in the long-term physical, cognitive, and emotional health and well-being of these fragile babies and their families.

SUMMARY

The disruption of normal brain growth and neurologic development is a significant consequence of preterm birth and can result in physical, emotional, and cognitive impairments. Improved survival rates for EP infants over recent decades have not yet been matched by clear evidence of a reduction in rates of neurodevelopmental disability. A high prevalence of intellectual disabilities, learning difficulties, and behavioral, social, and emotional problems continues to dominate the literature relating to childhood outcomes; recent reports have confirmed that these difficulties persist into adult life.

The persistence of neurodevelopmental sequelae from infancy to adulthood underscores the need for preventive intervention. Neuro-supportive and neuroprotective family centered developmental care is a preventive intervention for all preterm and EP infants. Such specialized care includes standardized care practices provided by a multidisciplinary team that has received education and training on the special needs of EP infants. This approach to care for this population of infants has shown to improve physical, cognitive, and emotional outcomes. For optimal neurodevelopmental outcomes, NICU staff should be experts in providing both clinical and neuroprotective support to babies as well as psychosocial support to parents and families.

REFERENCES

1. Anderson JG, Baer R, Partridge JC, et al. Survival and major morbidity of extremely preterm infants: a population-based study. Pediatrics 2016;138:138.
2. Lea C, Smith-Collins A, Luyt K. Protecting the premature brain: current evidence-based strategies for preventing perinatal brain injury in preterm infants. Arch Dis Child Fetal Neonatal Ed 2017;102:F176–82.
3. Costeloe K, Hennessy EM, Haider S, et al. Short-term outcomes after extreme preterm birth in England: comparison of two birth cohorts in 1995 and 2006 (the 32 EPICure studies). BMJ 2012;345:e7976.
4. Bockli K, Andrews B, Pellerite M, et al. Trends and challenges in the United States neonatal intensive care units follow-up clinics. J Perinatol 2014;34:71–4.
5. Altimier L, White R. The neonatal intensive care unit (NICU) environment. In: Kenner C, Lott J, editors. Comprehensive neonatal nursing care. New York: Springer Publishing; 2014. p. 722–38.

6. Altimier L, Phillips RM. The neonatal integrative developmental care model: seven neuroprotective core measures for family-centered developmental care. Newborn Infant Nurs Rev 2013;13(1):9–22.
7. Altimier L, Phillips RM. The neonatal integrative developmental care model: advanced clinical applications of the seven core measures for neuroprotective family-centered developmental care. Newborn Infant Nurs Rev 2016;16(4):230–44.
8. Bader L. Brain-oriented care in the NICU: a case study. Neonatal Netw 2014; 33(5):263–7.
9. Ditzenberger G, Blackburn S, Brown B, et al. Neurologic system. In: Kenner CL, Wright-Lott J, editors. Neonatal nursing care handbook: an evidence-based approach to conditions and procedures. New York: Springer Publishing Company; 2016. p. 83–172.
10. Dunn A. Brain challenge for premature babies. 2003. Available at: http://www.theage.com.au/articles/2003/11/28/1069825996785.html. Accessed August 30, 2018.
11. Hebb D. Foundations of psychological thought: a history of psychology. Oxford (England): Wiley; 1949.
12. Pickler R, McGrath JM, Reyna BA, et al. A model of neurodevelopmental risk and protection for preterm infants. J Perinat Neonatal Nurs 2010;24(4):356–65.
13. Bergman N. Skin-to-skin contact as a neurosupportive measure. Newborn Infant Nurs Rev 2015;15(3):145–50.
14. Bergman N. The neuroscience of birth – and the case for zero separation. Curationis 2014;37(2):1–4.
15. Bergman NJ. Neuroprotective core measures 1–7: neuroprotection of skin-to-skin contact (SSC). Newborn Infant Nurs Rev 2015;15(3):142–6.
16. Shonkoff JP. Building a new biodevelopmental framework to guide the future of early childhood policy. Child Dev 2010;81:357–67.
17. Bergman N, Linley LL, Fawcus SR. Randomized controlled trial of skin-to-skin contact from birth versus conventional incubator for physiological stabilization in 1200-2199 gram newborns. Acta Paediatr 2004;93(6):779–85.
18. Luong KC, Long Nguyen T, Thi H, et al. Newly born low birth weight infants stabilize better in skin-to-skin contact than when separated from their mothers: a randomized controlled trial. Acta Paediatr 2016;105(4):381–90.
19. Liao MC, Rao R, Mathur AM. Head position change is not associated with acute changes in bilateral cerebral oxygenation in stable preterm infants during the first 3 days of life. Am J Perinatol 2015;32(7):645–51.
20. Distefano G, Pratico AD. Actualities on molecular pathogenesis and repairing processes of cerebral damage in perinatal hypoxic-ischemic encephalopathy. Ital J Pediatr 2010;36:63.
21. Spittle A, Treyvaud K. The role of early developmental intervention to influence neurobehavioral outcomes of children born preterm. Semin Perinatol 2016; 40(8):542–8.
22. Doyle LW, Anderson PJ, Battin M, et al. Long term follow up of high risk children: who, why and how? BMC Pediatr 2014;14:279.
23. Anderson PJ, Cheong JL, Thompson DK. The predictive validity of neonatal MRI for neurodevelopmental outcome in very preterm children. Semin Perinatol 2015;39(2):147–58.
24. Smith GC, Gutovich J, Smyser C, et al. Neonatal intensive care unit stress is associated with brain development in preterm infants. Ann Neurol 2011;70(4):541–9.
25. Rabe H, Diaz-Rossello JL, Duley L, et al. Effect of timing of umbilical cord clamping and other strategies to influence placental transfusion at preterm

birth on maternal and infant outcomes. Cochrane Database Syst Rev 2012;(8):CD003248.
26. Backes C, Rivera BK, Haque U, et al. Placental transfusion strategies in very preterm neonates: a systematic review and meta-analysis. Obstet Gynecol 2014;124:47–56.
27. Brocato B, Holliday N, Whitehurst RM Jr, et al. Delayed cord clamping in preterm neonates: a review of benefits and risks. Obstet Gynecol Surv 2016;71:39–42.
28. Fowlie P, Davis PG, McGuire W. Prophylactic intravenous indomethacin for preventing mortality and morbidity in preterm infants. Cochrane Database Syst Rev 2010;(7):CD003248.
29. Ballabh P. Pathogenesis and prevention of intraventricular hemorrhage. Clin Perinatol 2014;41:47–67.
30. Ment L, Vohr B, Allan W, et al. Outcome of children in the indomethacin intraventricular hemorrhage prevention trial. Pediatrics 2000;105:485–91.
31. Morton S, Smith V. Treatment options for apnoea of prematurity. Arch Dis Child Fetal Neonatal Ed 2016;101(4):F352–6.
32. Henderson-Smart DJ, De Paoli AG. Methylxanthine treatment for apnoea in preterm infants. Cochrane Database Syst Rev 2010;(140):CD003248.
33. Schmidt B, Roberts RS, Davis P, et al. Long-term effects of caffeine therapy for apnea of prematurity. N Engl J Med 2007;357:1893–902.
34. McPherson C, Neil JJ, Tjoeng TH, et al. A pilot randomized trial of high-dose caffeine therapy in preterm infants. Pediatr Res 2015;78:198–204.
35. Dobson N, Patel RM, Smith PB, et al. Trends in caffeine use and association between clinical outcomes and timing of therapy in very low birth weight infants. J Pediatr 2014;164:992–8.
36. Heuchan A, Clyman RI. Managing the patent ductus arteriosus: current treatment options. Arch Dis Child Fetal Neonatal Ed 2014;99:F431–6.
37. Hamrick S, Hansmann G. Patent ductus arteriosus of the preterm infant. Pediatrics 2010;125(1020–1030):1020.
38. Evans N. Preterm patent ductus arteriosus: a continuing conundrum for the neonatologist? Semin Fetal Neonatal Med 2015;20:272–7.
39. Kluckow M, Jeffery M, Gill A, et al. A randomised placebo-controlled trial of early treatment of the patent ductus arteriosus. Arch Dis Child Fetal Neonatal Ed 2014;99:F99–104.
40. Mitha A, Foix-L'Helias L, Arnaud C, et al. Neonatal infection and 5-year neurodevelopmental outcome of very preterm infants. Pediatrics 2013;132:E372–80.
41. Adams-Chapman I. Long-term impact of infection on the preterm neonate. Semin Perinatol 2012;36:462–70.
42. Rand K, Austin NC, Inder TE, et al. Neonatal infection and later neurodevelopmental risk in the very preterm infant. J Pediatr 2016;170:97–104.
43. Hentges CR, Silveira RC, Procianoy RS, et al. Association of late-onset neonatal sepsis with late neurodevelopment in the first two years of life of preterm infants with very low birth weight. J Pediatr 2014;90:50–7.
44. Stoll BJ, Hansen NI, Adams-Chapman I, et al. Neurodevelopmental and growth impairment among extremely low-birth-weight infants with neonatal infection. JAMA 2004;292:2357–65.
45. Shane AL, Komenda P. Neonatal sepsis: progress towards improved outcomes. J Infect 2014;68(S1):S24–32.
46. Davis J, Odd D, Jary S, et al. The impact of a sepsis quality improvement project on neurodisability rates in very low birthweight infants. Arch Dis Child Fetal Neonatal Ed 2016;101:F562–4.

47. Cortez J, Makker K, Kraemer DF, et al. Maternal milk feedings reduce sepsis, necrotizing enterocolitis and improve outcomes of premature infants. J Perinatol 2018;38(1):71–4.
48. Aceti A, Maggio L, Beghetti I, et al. Probiotics prevent late-onset sepsis in human milk-fed, very low birth weight preterm infants: systematic review and meta-analysis. Nutrients 2017;9(8):904.
49. Romagnoli C. Risk factors and growth factors in ROP. Early Hum Dev 2009; 85(10 Suppl):S79–82.
50. Manzoni P, Stolfi I, Pedicino R, et al. Human milk feeding prevents retinopathy of prematurity (ROP) in preterm VLBW neonates. Early Hum Dev 2013;89:S64–8.
51. Gilbert C, Wormald R, Fielder A, et al. Potential for a paradigm change in the detection of retinopathy of prematurity requiring treatment. Arch Dis Child Fetal Neonatal Ed 2016;101:F6.
52. Schanler RJ, Lau C, Hurst NM, et al. Randomized trial of donor human milk versus preterm formula as substitutes for mothers' own milk in the feeding of extremely premature infants. Pediatrics 2005;116(2):400–6.
53. Zhou J, Shukla VV, John D, et al. Human milk feeding as a protective factor for retinopathy of prematurity: A meta-analysis. Pediatrics 2015;136:e1576–86.
54. Ginovart G, Gich I, Verd S. Human milk feeding protects very low-birth-weight infants from retinopathy of prematurity: A pre–post cohort analysis. J. Matern-Fetal Neonatal Med 2016;29:3790–5.
55. Miller J, Tonkin E, Damarell RA, et al. A Systematic Review and Meta-Analysis of Human Milk Feeding and Morbidity in Very Low Birth Weight Infants. Nutrients 2018;10(6):707. https://doi.org/10.3390/nu10060707.
56. Hylander MA, Strobino DM, Pezzullo JC, et al. Association of human milk feedings with a reduction in retinopathy of prematurity among very low birthweight infants. J Perinatol 2001;21(6):356–62.
57. Lynch A, Wagner B, Hodges J, et al. The relationship of the subtypes of preterm birth with retinopathy of prematurity. Am J Obstet Gynecol 2017;217(3):354.e1–8.
58. Cayabyab R, Arora V, Wertheimer F, et al. Graded oxygen saturation targets and retinopathy of prematurity in extremely preterm infants. Pediatric Research 2016;80(3):401–6.
59. Nathan A, Ward L, Schibler K, et al. A quality improvement initiative to reduce necrotizing enterocolitis across hospital systems. J Perinatol 2018;38(6):742–50.
60. Martin CR, Dammann O, Allred EN, et al. Neurodevelopment of extremely preterm infants who had necrotizing enterocolitis with or without late bacteremia. J Pediatr 2010;157:751–6.
61. Shah DK, Dammann O, Anderson PJ, et al. Adverse neurodevelopment in preterm infants with postnatal sepsis or necrotizing enterocolitis is mediated by white matter abnormalities on magnetic resonance imaging at term. J Pediatr 2008;153:170–5.
62. Lodha A, Seshia M, McMillan D, et al. Association of early caffeine administration and neonatal outcomes in very preterm neonates. JAMA Pediatr 2015;169(1):33–8.
63. Wadhawan R, Oh W, Hintz SR, et al. Neurodevelopmental outcomes of extremely low birth weight infants with spontaneous intestinal perforation or surgical necrotizing enterocolitis. J Perinatol 2014;34:64–70.
64. Hintz SR, Kendrick DE, Wilson-Costello DE, et al. Early-childhood neurodevelopmental outcomes are not improving for infants born at <25 weeks' gestational age. Pediatrics 2011;127(1):62–70.
65. Embleton ND, Zalewski S, Berrington JE. Probiotics for prevention of necrotizing enterocolitis and sepsis in preterm infants. Curr Opin Infect Dis 2016;29:256–61.

66. Pammi M, Abrams SA. Oral lactoferrin for the prevention of sepsis and necrotizing enterocolitis in preterm infants. Cochrane Database Syst Rev 2015;(2):CD007137.
67. Sisk PM, Lovelady CA, Dillard RG, et al. Early human milk feeding is associated with a lower risk of necrotizing enterocolitis in very low birth weight infants. J Perinatol 2007;27:428–33.
68. Battersby C, Longford N, Mandalia S, et al. Incidence and enteral feed antecedents of severe neonatal necrotising enterocolitis across neonatal networks in England, 2012-13: a whole-population surveillance study. Lancet Gastroenterol Hepatol 2016;2:43–51.
69. Lin HC, Su BH, Chen AC, et al. Oral probiotics reduce the incidence and severity of necrotizing enterocolitis in very low birth weight infants. Pediatrics 2005;115:1–4.
70. Meinzen-Derr J, Poindexter B, Wrage L, et al. Role of human milk in extremely low birth weight infants' risk of necrotizing enterocolitis or death. J Perinatol 2009;29:1–5.
71. Als H, Duffy FH, McAnulty GB, et al. Early experience alters brain function and structure. Pediatrics 2004;113(4):846–57.
72. Vohr BR, Poindexter BB, Dusick AM, et al. Beneficial effects of breast milk in the neonatal intensive care unit on the developmental outcome of extremely low birth weight infants at 18 months of age. Pediatrics 2006;118:E115–23.
73. Belfort MB, Anderson PJ, Nowak PJ, et al. Breast milk feeding, brain development, and neurocognitive outcomes: a 7-year longitudinal study in infants born at less than 30 weeks' gestation. J Pediatr 2016;177:133–9.
74. Su BH. Optimizing nutrition in preterm infants. Pediatr Neonatol 2014;55:5–13.
75. Isaacs E, Fischl BR, Quinn BT, et al. Impact of breast milk on intelligence quotient, brain size, and white matter development. Pediatr Res 2010;67(4):357–62.
76. Sammallahti S, Kajantie E, Matinolli H-M, et al. Nutrition after preterm birth and adult neurocognitive outcomes. PLoS One 2017;12:e0185632.
77. Schanler R. Outcomes of Human Milk-Fed Premature Infants. Seminars in Perinatology 2011;35(1):29–33.
78. Horbar JD, Badger GJ, Lewit EM, et al, Vermont Oxford Network. Hospital and patient characteristics associated with variation in 28-day mortality rates for very low birth weight infants. Pediatrics 1997;99(2):149–56.
79. Lee SK, McMillan DD, Ohlsson A, et al. Variations in practice and outcomes in the Canadian NICU network: 1996-1997. Pediatrics 2000;106(5):1070–9.
80. Vohr BR, Wright LL, Dusick AM, et al, Neonatal Research Network. Center differences and outcomes of extremely low birth weight infants. Pediatrics 2004; 113(4):781–9.
81. Improvement, I.o.H. PDSA Cycle. 2016. Available at: http://www.ihi.org/resources/Pages/HowtoImprove/ScienceofImprovementHowtoImprove.aspx. Accessed August 30, 2018.
82. Aziz K, McMillan DD, Andrews W, et al. Variations in rates of nosocomial infection among Canadian neonatal intensive care units may be practice-related. BMC Pediatr 2005;5(1):22–34.
83. Chow L, Wright KW, Sola A, CSMC Oxygen Administration Study Group. Can changes in clinical practice decrease the incidence of severe retinopathy of prematurity in very low birth weight infants? Pediatrics 2003;111(2):339–45.
84. Payne NR, Finkelstein MJ, Liu M, et al. NICU practices and outcomes associated with 9 years of quality improvement collaboratives. Pediatrics 2010;125(3):437–46.

85. Levesque BM, Kalish LA, LaPierre J, et al. Impact of implementing 5 potentially better respiratory practices on neonatal outcomes and costs. Pediatrics 2011; 128(1):e218–26.
86. Schmutz J, Manser T. Do team processes really have an effect on clinical performance? A systematic literature review. Br J Anaesth 2013;110(4): 529–44.
87. Salas E, Rosen MA. Building high reliability teams: progress and some reflections on teamwork training. BMJ Qual Saf 2013;22(5):369–73.
88. Nankervis C, Martin EM, Crane ML, et al. Implementation of a multidisciplinary guideline-driven approach to the care of the extremely premature infant improved hospital outcomes. Acta Paediatr 2010;99(2):188–93.
89. Morris M, Cleary J, Soliman A. Small baby unit improves quality and outcomes in extremely low birth weight infants. Pediatrics 2015;136(4):E1007–101.
90. Altimier L, et al. Developmental care: changing the nicu physically and behaviorally to promote patient outcomes and contain costs. Neonatal Intensive Care 2005;18(4):12–6.
91. Altimier L, Kenner C, Damus K. The effect of a comprehensive developmental care training program: wee care neuroprotective program (wee care) on seven neuroprotective core measures for family-centered developmental care of premature neonates. Newborn Infant Nurs Rev 2015;15(1):6–16.
92. Hendricks-Muñoz K, et al. Developmental care: the impact of wee care developmental care training on short-term infant outcome and hospital costs. Newborn Infant Nurs Rev 2002;2(1):39–45.
93. Ludwig S, et al. Quality improvement analysis of developmental care in infants less than 1500 grams at birth. Newborn Infant Nurs Rev 2008;8(2):94–100.
94. Phillips RM. Seven core measures of neuroprotective family-centered developmental care: creating an infrastructure for implementation. Newborn Infant Nurs Rev 2015;15(3):4.
95. Als H. NIDCAP: testing the effectiveness of a relationship-based comprehensive intervention. Pediatrics 2009;124(4):1208–10.
96. Sharek P, Powers R, Koehn A, et al. Evaluation and development of potentially better practices to improve pain management of neonates. Pediatrics 2006; 118(Suppl 2):S78–86.
97. Greene M, Rossman B, Patra K, et al. Depression, anxiety, and perinatal-specific posttraumatic distress in mothers of very low birth weight infants in the neonatal intensive care unit. J Dev Behav Pediatr 2015;36(5):362–70.
98. Hynan M, Hall S. Psychosocial program standards for NICU parents. J Perinatol 2015;35(S1-S4):S1.
99. Association, N.P. Support 4 NICU parents. 2018. Available at: http://support4nicuparents.org/. Accessed August 30, 2018.
100. Hall S, Mosher S, Sorrells K. My NICU Network. 2018. Available at: http://www.mynicunetwork.com/. Accessed August 30, 2018.
101. Cooper LG, Gooding JS,, Gallagher J, et al. Impact of family-centered care initiative on NICU care, staff and families. J Perinatol 2007;27:S32–7.
102. Als H, Lawhon G, Duffy FH, et al. Individualized developmental care for the very-low-birth-weight preterm infant:Medical and neurofunctional effects. JAMA 1994;272:853–8.
103. Melnyk BM, Feinstein NF, Alpert-Gillis L, et al. Reducing premature infants' length of stay and improving parents' mental health outcomes with the Creating Opportunities for Parent Empowerment (COPE) neonatal intensive

care unit program: a randomized, controlled trial. Pediatrics 2006;111(5): e1414–27.

104. Johnson S, Marlow N. Early and long-term outcome of infants born extremely preterm. Arch Dis Child 2016;102(1):97–102.

105. Degos V, Loron G, Mantz J, et al. Neuroprotective strategies for the neonatal brain. Anesth Analg 2008;106:1670–80.

APPENDIX 1: NEONATAL INTEGRATIVE DEVELOPMENTAL CARE MODEL: *QUICK TIPS* TO IMPLEMENT THE 7 CORE MEASURES FOR NEUROPROTECTIVE FAMILY-CENTERED DEVELOPMENTAL CARE

Guiding principles

- All infants are in a critical period of brain growth and organization.
  - Everything that happens in the NICU impacts brain development.
  - Providing excellent, evidence-based medical care is always our goal.
  - The *way* we provide our care influences developmental outcomes.
- Neuroprotective developmental care is relational.
  - Treat every infant as a little human being who has his or her own unique identity.
  - Speak directly to the infant in soft tones to tell him or her what is happening.
  - Do examinations and procedures *with* the infant, not *to* the infant.
  - Notice individual differences and preferences in each infant.
- Emotional connection with parents/families is essential for optimal outcomes.
  - Parents are the most important caregivers for their infant in the long run.
  - Support parent-infant attachment in every possible way in the NICU.
  - Provide psychosocial support for NICU parents as needed.
- SSC is the most fundamental form of neuroprotective care.
  - SSC with the mother is the natural habitat for all newborn infants outside the womb.
  - SSC supports all 7 of the neuroprotective core measures.
  - Encourage/facilitate early and prolonged SSC whenever possible.

Core measure 1: healing environment

A healing environment protects the developing sensory system of preterm infants.

- Protect the tactile system with gentle touch.
  - Provide gentle yet firm tactile support.
  - Facilitate early, frequent, and prolonged SSC.
  - Promote infant massage when appropriate.
- Protect the vestibular system with slow movements.
  - Use slow, gentle movements during handling.
  - Contain the infant in all care (positioning, bathing, weighing, holding, and so forth).
  - Eliminate moving infants to different bed-spaces to accommodate staffing patterns.
- Protect the olfactory system by minimizing odors.
  - Let hand sanitizers dry before putting hands inside incubator.
  - Maintain a fragrance-free and scent-free NICU.
  - Expose infant to mother's scent when possible via breast pad, or soft cloth.
- Protect the gustatory system by providing positive taste opportunities.
  - Provide breastmilk mouth care.
  - Promote nuzzling/suckling when SSC.
  - Position infant with hands near face.

- Protect the auditory system by minimizing noise.
  - Talk in a library voice when near bedsides.
  - Keep pagers and phones on vibrate.
  - Noise meters/red/yellow/green traffic lights should be set 55 dB or less.
- Protect the visual system by minimizing direct light.
  - Cover the infant's eyes during examinations and procedures.
  - Be sure the incubator covers and blankets protect from direct light.
  - Use diurnal lighting for infants greater than 31 weeks' Corrected Gestational Age (CGA).

Core measure 2: partnering with families

Parents are the most important caregivers in an infant's life.

- Go out of your way to make parents feel welcome in the NICU.
  - Always greet parents and introduce yourself with your name and role.
  - Having an infant in the NICU is usually an unexpected crisis for families.
  - Expect the need to repeat conversations/explanations more than once.
  - Use lay language free from acronyms when talking with parents.
- Involve parents as active members of the caregiving team.
  - Educate, coach, and mentor parents in caring for their infant in the NICU.
  - Include parents in medical rounds and nursing shift change discussions.
  - Ask parents how they think their infant is doing, and then listen.
- SSC helps heal the wounds of interrupted bonding and attachment.
  - Recognize the importance of parent-infant attachment on brain development.
  - Facilitate early, frequent, and prolonged SSC.

Core measure 3: positioning and handling

Positioning should mimic the fetal position in the womb.

- Maintain the head in a midline position.
  - Be extra vigilant with ventilated ELBW infants.
  - Ask the Respiratory Care Provider (RCP) to help reposition endotracheal tube and/or reposition the infant if needed.
- Maintain the limbs and trunk in flexed, tucked position.
  - Gently reposition the infant after extending limbs during examinations/procedures.
  - Reposition the infant in a positioning aid after examinations/procedures.
- Handle preterm and sick infants with slow, gentle movements.
  - Ask for help with procedures or complicated handling.
  - Ask staff or parents to provide 4-handed support if needed.
  - Monitor the infant closely during interventions for behavioral cues that indicate stress.
- SSC is the natural habitat for all newborn infants.
  - SSC is the closest to being back inside the womb.
  - Facilitate early, frequent, and prolonged SSC.

Core measure 4: safeguarding sleep

Sleep is essential for healing, growth, and optimal brain development.

- Never waken a sleeping infant unless necessary.
  - Support long periods of restful, uninterrupted sleep whenever possible.
  - Time routine cares/examinations to coincide with the infant's sleep/wake cycles.
  - Wake the infant slowly, gently, with a soft voice associated with touch.

- Protect sleep states by minimizing noise and light.
  - Talk in a library voice when near bedsides.
  - Be sure direct light is not shining on sleeping infants.
- Group interventions (assessments, laboratory tests, vital signs, and so forth) to provide long periods of undisturbed rest.
  - Continuous evaluation during these groupings is essential to ensure the infant is tolerating the procedures and is not overly stressed.
  - Monitor the infant's ability to self-calm.
- SSC promotes the most optimal sleep cycles.
  - Remember, newborn infants sleep best when in SSC.
  - Facilitate early, frequent, and prolonged SSC.

Core measure 5: minimizing stress and pain

Stress and pain are part of NICU life, but both can be minimized.

- Supporting a healing environment helps to minimize stress.
  - Protect infants from excess noise and light.
  - Talk in a library voice and cover the infant's eyes during examinations.
  - Watch for signs of stress during examinations, and pause when possible.
  - Extended digits and limbs indicate stress.
  - Excessive tone or absence of tone indicates stress.
- Use positioning and boundaries to provide containment.
  - Be sure the infant is well contained during examinations and procedures.
  - Be sure the infant is repositioned properly after examinations and procedures.
- Use extra supports during painful procedures.
  - Ask staff or parents to provide 4-handed support when needed.
  - Many parents are willing and eager to help support their baby.
  - Give them a chance to participate if they are available and willing.
- Be sure Sweet-Ease is given 2 minutes before painful procedures.
  - Understand the mechanism of action (activation of endogenous opioid receptors).
  - Understand absorption (via buccal mucosa, not via digestion).
- Be sure adequate analgesics are given for painful procedures if needed.
  - Be proactive with postoperative pain management.
- SSC reduces stress and pain; the mother's presence is analgesic.
  - Facilitate early, frequent, and prolonged SSC.

Core measure 6: protecting skin

Skin is a conduit for nerve cells to send sensory messages to the brain.

- Monitor the humidity level inside the incubator during first week for ELBW infants
  - Be sure humidity is provided until skin is keratinized, about 5 to 10 days.
    - Being skin to skin on mother's chest provides about 50% humidity.
- Monitor nasal septum for skin breakdown if nasal prongs are used.
  - Check prongs frequently; there should be no pressure on the septum.
  - Check the septum each shift for erythema or breakdown.
- Monitor other susceptible skin areas.
  - Check the mouth for oral thrush and the diaper area for rash.
  - Check trunk/limbs for pressure ulcers and IV sites for erythema/infiltrates.
- Provide education to families on how to do swaddled bathing.
- Provide a quiet, dim, draft-free environment.
- Provide a radiant warm heat source to promote a neutral-thermal environment.

Core measure 7: optimizing nutrition

Human milk is the optimal diet for most human infants.

- Discuss the medical need for breastmilk with parents whenever the opportunity arises.
  - Explain how breastmilk is a medicine, especially for preterm infants.
  - Explain the need for early/frequent pumping if the infant is unable to breastfeed.
- Support the mother's early and continued milk supply.
  - Provide enthusiastic support for any breastmilk the mother provides.
  - Explain the importance of ongoing pumping to maintain milk supply.
- Provide ongoing breastfeeding education and support.
  - Explain how important breastmilk is for healing and nutrition.
  - Explain how important breastmilk is for brain development and vision.
  - Explain how important breastmilk is to decrease the risk of NEC and sepsis.
- SSC increases breastfeeding initiation and duration.
  - SSC increases prolactin and oxytocin, both needed for lactation.
  - Facilitate early, frequent, and prolonged SSC.
- Cue-based, infant-driven feeding prevents later oral aversions.
  - Oral feedings should be safe, developmentally appropriate, and nurturing.
  - Provide cue-based rather than volume feedings.
  - Monitor feeding readiness and signs of stress during feeds.
- Support breastfeeding well before discharge.
  - Infants can practice suckling when skin to skin whenever interested.
  - The first oral feeding should be at the breast if the mother has been pumping.
  - If a term infant has difficulty latching, provide lactation consultant support.
  - Check mouth for anomalies, for example, cleft (cleft palate or tongue-tie).
  - If anomalies are present, alert physician to get appropriate treatment.
  - Create a feeding plan with the NICU nutrition specialist that includes breastfeeding at home in addition to fortified bottle feeds if needed.
  - Provide the mother with community resources for breastfeeding support.

From Altimier L, Phillips R. The neonatal integrative developmental care model: advanced clinical applications of the seven core measures for neuroprotective family-centered developmental care. Newborn Infant Nurs Rev 2016;16(4):242; with permission.

APPENDIX 2: SMALL BABY PROGRAM: DAILY CHECKLIST FOR THE FIRST 72 HOURS AT 23- TO 29-WEEKS' GESTATION (REVIEW CHECKLIST WITH CARE TEAM DURING DAILY ROUNDS)

	Reason Incomplete
Partnering with families Educate, coach, and mentor parents in becoming active participants in their infant's care in supporting their infant's developmental goals. Encourage zero separation between parents and infant. • Support families with a warm, respectful, and welcoming manner. • Focus on parents' emotional connection with the infant when parents first arrive at bedside each day. • Orient parents regarding good hand hygiene and cleanliness of the NICU environment. • Provide family frequent, timely, and accurate information (provide admission information). • Introduce parents to care team and encourage parents to participate in rounds and hand-offs. • Begin teaching how to do simple care, such as taking temperature or providing hand support during care. • Facilitate early, frequent, and prolonged SSC.	
Healing environment Educate, coach, and mentor parents on the importance of creating a healing environment that protects the developing sensory system of the preterm infant. Emphasize their central role in the healing environment as parents and as active members of the caregiving team. • Keep touch, movement, odors, negative oral stimuli, noise, and direct light to a minimum; cover incubator. • Introduce parents to the purpose and use of scent cloth (olfactory support). • Minimize negative perioral stimulation (adhesives, suctioning, and so forth); promote positive oral stimulation, cue-based non-nutritive sucking, with hands supported near face. • Silence alarms as quickly as possible; turn phones and beepers to vibrate. • Protect eyes during exposure to direct light.	
Positioning and handling Educate, coach, and mentor parents on how to developmentally position, handle, and contain their infant. • Position the bed so that infant can be approached from both sides and with the head of bed up 20° to 30°. • Position the head midline in neutral positioning (supine or side lying only). • Use therapeutic positioning aids to maintain alignment, flexion, containment, and boundaries circumferentially (360°). • Promote hands to mouth/face contact. • Handle gently with slow movements with position changes and care activities, using 2-person/4-handed support.	
Safeguarding sleep Educate, coach, and mentor parents on sleep-wake states and how to promote sleep in their infant. • Avoid sleep interruptions from loud noises, bright lights, and unnecessary disturbing activities. • Protect infant's eyes from direct light exposure and maintain low levels of ambient light.	

(*continued on next page*)

(continued)	Reason Incomplete
• Individualize all caregiving activities by clustering care based on infant sleep-wake states. Take care not to overstress the infant with too many clustered cares at once. • If it is necessary to arouse a sleeping infant, approach using a soft voice/whisper followed by gentle touch. • Schedule touch times every 4 to 6 hours and as needed.	
Minimizing stress and pain Educate, coach, and mentor parents on infant cues related to stress and pain and how to provide their infant with nonpharmacologic support during stressful or painful procedures. • Provide nonpharmacologic support (breast milk, SSC, sucrose, pacifier) with all minor invasive interventions • Support daily NICU quiet time. • Provide guidance to parents on how to collaborate with NICU staff to minimize their baby's stress & pain • Evaluate clinical need for all laboratory tests/tests/procedures and reduce number of stressful/painful laboratory tests/tests/procedures when possible • Gently draw laboratory tests as ordered using nonpharmacologic support and using 2-person/4-handed support.	
Protecting skin Educate, coach, and mentor parents on how to protect their infant's skin and its many functions, including its role as a conduit of neurosensory information to the brain. • Use servo-control to provide neutral thermal environment, keeping the incubator closed as much as possible. • Provide 70% to 85% humidity for the first 7 days of life; if condensation forms, decrease 5% every hour until it is gone. • If on noninvasive support, ensure correct prong/hat size and face placement to protect skin integrity. • Minimize the use of adhesives and use caution when removing adhesives to prevent epidermal stripping. • Defer bath for first 72 hours and until the skin is not gelatinous; providing rationale to parents.	
Optimizing nutrition: fluids, electrolytes, nutrition Educate, coach, and mentor parents about the importance of mother's own breast milk as a medicine for their infant. (if breast milk is used) • Use central IV access (UVC and UAC preferred or PICC). • Maintain total fluids ordered (including TPN, Intralipids (IL), feedings, IV flushes and medications) at ordered mL/kg/d. • Weigh the infant daily inside positioning supports and calibrate the scale with positioning support (bunting/snuggle), diaper, and hat. • Educate the mother about hand expression, the use of colostrum, pumping, and expressed breast milk supply. • Initiate feeds of human milk (mother's own or donor) using feeding protocol.	
Respiratory • If intubated, monitor the ETT position and securement, always maintaining the head in midline alignment. • If on non-invasive ventilation, monitor position of nasal apparatus to maintain functional residual capacity (FRC) and provide appropriately sized head gear for comfort and to prevent head molding. • Set pulse oximeter alarm limits (low limit 90%, high limit 96%) or per order.	

(continued on next page)

(continued)	
	Reason Incomplete
Other monitoring, medications, and IV fluids • Start caffeine on day of life 1 to 2; schedule the caffeine maintenance dose to begin 24 hours after the loading dose. • Perform oral care with colostrum when available and breast milk when there is no colostrum. • Administer antibiotics as ordered. • Consider vitamin A administration. • Consider NIRS/aEEG.	

Abbreviations: aEEG, amplitude-integrated electroencephalogram; ETT, endotracheal tube; NIRS, near-infrared spectroscopy; PICC, peripherally inserted central catheters; TPN, total parenteral nutrition; UAC, umbilical artery catheter; UVC, umbilical venous catheter.

[illegible]

Neonatal Abstinence Syndrome: An Uncontrollable Epidemic

Nancy J. MacMullen, PhD, APN/CNS, RNC, HR-OB, CNE*,
Linda F. Samson, PhD, RN, BC, NEA, BC[1]

KEYWORDS

- Neonatal abstinence syndrome • Intensive care unit • Drug withdrawal
- Opioid abuse • Evidence based nursing interventions

KEY POINTS

- Neonatal abstinence syndrome (NAS) admissions are increasing due to an upsurge in opioid use among pregnant women.
- Nursing interventions for infants with NAS must be evidence based.
- Options for clinical management include pharmacologic intervention, alternative therapy, and family interventions.
- Interventions begin with the mother no matter what stage of the reproductive cycle she is in.
- Surveillance and prevention are important concepts in caring for mothers who are drug dependent.

Currently, there is an escalation of drug abuse in the global population. The United Nations Office on Drugs and Crime in the 2017 World Drug Report[1] states that 29.5% of the global adult population suffers from drug abuse disorders. The organization includes opioid abuse in the report and identifies opioids and their derivatives as the most harmful of the drugs abused.[1] The opioid epidemic has likewise affected the United States and has health professionals and health care agencies alarmed. The increased dependency on this drug is a growing problem that affects persons of all ages. Opioid drugs abused by childbearing women, however, who then may become pregnant are of special concern. The effects of the drug use and withdrawal affect not

Disclosure: The authors have nothing to disclose.
Department of Nursing, Governors State University, 1 University Parkway, University Park, IL 60484, USA
[1] Present address: 1860 Waterford Court, Highland, Park, IL 60035.
* Corresponding author. 5948 Liberty Square, Oak Forest, IL 60452
E-mail address: nmacmullen@govst.edu

Crit Care Nurs Clin N Am 30 (2018) 585–596
https://doi.org/10.1016/j.cnc.2018.07.011 ccnursing.theclinics.com

1 but 2 people: the mother and the fetus. The syndrome of infant withdrawal from opioids is called neonatal abstinence syndrome (NAS).[2]

PURPOSE

The incidence of NAS has increased substantially in the past decade.[3] Neonates with NAS often require specialized care in the neonatal ICU (NICU). Caring for a neonate with NAS, which may be coupled with other neonatal complications, such as prematurity, presents a unique challenge to nurses working with these special neonates. The purpose of this article is to thoroughly discuss NAS and to determine what strategies are available to control an uncontrollable epidemic of the syndrome. Evidence-based interventions for neonatal nursing practice are emphasized.

DEFINITION

NAS is a drug withdrawal syndrome that occurs in primarily opioid-exposed neonates after birth often with central nervous system and gastrointestinal symptoms.[4] The definition of NAS has been expanded by some professionals in the field to include other drugs besides opioids (cocaine, amphetamines, and barbiturates).[3] The term NAS in this article is the classic/original definition—neonatal withdrawal from opioids.[4]

INCIDENCE

Illicit Drugs

Use of illicit drugs (including opioids) in general is a problem for pregnant women, who are cautioned to avoid harmful substances that may result in perinatal complications. The report, "Results from the 2013 National Survey on Drug Use and Health: Summary of National Findings," indicates that the rate of illicit drug use among pregnant women in the United States aged 15 to 44 averaged across 2012 and 2013 was 5.4%. The rate for pregnant women aged 15 to 17 was 14.6%. It was 8.6% among women aged 18 to 25 and 3.2% among women aged 26 to 44.[5] These results were not significantly different from data from 2010 to 2011. International data for the comparable period show 4.2% of Australian women overall consuming illicit drugs, a much lower rate than in the United States.[6]

Opioids

Abuse of opioid drugs in the United States has increased dramatically, affecting the lives of thousands of people. A statistical brief of the Healthcare Cost and Utilization Project states that opioid overdoses (prescription opiates and illicit opioids) have increased 200% and has been declared an opioid epidemic by the US Department of Health and Human Services.[7]

Neonatal Abstinence Syndrome

Along with the rise of opioid use and abuse, there was a concomitant increase in the occurrence of NAS.[3] The overall incidence of NAS in the United States grew approximately 300% during the years 1999 to 2013.[8] Admissions of neonates with NAS to NICUs surged. From 2004 to 2013, admissions to the unit escalated from 7 cases per 1000 admissions to 27 cases per 1000 admissions, with an increase in the median length of stay from 13 days to 19 days.[9] Overall incidence of NAS ranges from 48% to 94% in infants born to mothers who are abusing substances at the time of delivery in data collected from a Cochrane review.[10]

DIAGNOSIS

Maternal History

A diagnosis of NAS is accomplished through taking a thorough taking maternal history and performing a detailed, systematic, physical assessment of the neonate. A clinician presents the items in the maternal history in a nonjudgmental manner, because the woman may be reluctant to communicate information that may have legal and ethical consequences.[3] Maternal history includes the onset, duration, types, amount of the drug(s), time of the last dose, duration of exposure, the total accumulation of exposure, and the number of substances to which the neonate was exposed.[11]

Neonatal Assessment

Diagnosis of NAS is one of evaluation of signs and symptoms of opioid withdrawal. All neonates born to mothers who used opiates during the pregnancy are monitored for signs and symptoms of NAS for 5 days minimally to determine the necessity for treatment.[12] Diagnostic signs and symptoms include extreme irritability, excessive and high-pitched crying, sleep disturbances, failure to self-soothe, and increased muscle tone tremors and seizures. Other signs and symptoms that may be observed are diarrhea, abnormal heart and respiratory rates, temperature instability, mottling, sweating, and yawning[13] (**Table 1**).

Assessment Instruments

Clinical instruments, such as the Finnegan Neonatal Abstinence Scoring Tool, have been developed and used in the diagnosis of NAS and aid in the objective assessment of these neonates. The Finnegan is the most widely used and is available in the original or modified version.[3] The instrument has a 5-point scale to rate the signs and symptoms of the various organ systems involved in NAS: gastrointestinal, metabolic, vasomotor, central nervous system (CNS), and respiratory at birth and every 4 hours after feeding.[13] There are 30 items across 21 categories, with a minimum score of 0 and a maximum score of 44.[14] The more severe the symptoms, the higher the score. Although the Finnegan instrument is the most widely used, there are other clinical assessment instruments available. They include the MOTHER (Maternal Opioid Treatment Experimental Research) NAS scale, the Lipsitz Neonatal Drug Withdrawal Scoring System, and the Neonatal Withdrawal Inventory. All the instruments can be used to aid in clinical decision making and initiating treatment.[14]

Table 1
Signs and symptoms of neonatal abstinence syndrome in the neonate

System	Signs and Symptoms
CNS	Irritability, jitteriness, tremors, and excessive crying Hyperirritability leads to agitation, difficulty sleeping, and inconsolable crying High-pitched cry
Autonomic nervous system	Impaired heart rate, respiratory rate, and muscle tone Temperature instability, sweating, mottling, and sneezing
Respiratory system	Tachypnea, nasal flaring, nasal stuffiness
Gastrointestinal system	Poor feeding, regurgitation, vomiting, and diarrhea

Data from Kocherlakota P. Neonatal abstinence syndrome. Pediatrics 2014;134(2):e547–61.

Laboratory Analysis

Although the assessment instruments are used for the clinical diagnosis, laboratory tests are necessary to identify and confirm the type of substance abused by the mother. Analysis of a neonate's meconium or urine is done as screening tests with confirmatory diagnosis accomplished by mass spectrometry.[11] A multimethod approach, which includes identification of neonates at risk for NAS via maternal history of drug abuse, screening instruments, and laboratory tests of maternal and fetal biologic specimens, is recommended as is a protocol for newborn screening.[3]

CLINICAL MANAGEMENT

There have been numerous strategies for the clinical management of neonates suffering from NAS depending on the severity of symptoms, infant birthweight, and, in some cases, the research that is being conducted at the particular center where care is being delivered. The most frequently used protocol still provides opioids to the infant based on the Finnegan NAS scoring system, modified Finnegan NAS scoring system, or one of the other tools previously described.[3,14–17] To provide a comprehensive discussion of current clinical management approaches, the article addresses pharmacologic interventions, alternative therapy, and family therapy with the rationale for each of the approaches.

Pharmacologic Intervention

Pharmacologic intervention includes administration of any one of the opioid or opioid derivative drugs to combat the neonatal withdrawal from the maternal opioid drugs that have been present in the fetus prior to delivery and in the neonate after birth. According to Brown and colleagues,[18] and review of the American Academy of Pediatrics guidelines, 2012, that were reaffirmed in February of 2016,[19] when pharmacologic intervention is required after failure of nonpharmacologic intervention, the primary treatment is usually with either morphine or methadone. A list of pharmacologic agents in current use is included in **Table 2**.[11]

Morphine is often the first-line drug used when scoring guidelines suggest the need for pharmacologic intervention.[18,20–23] Recent studies suggest that administration of methadone may lead to earlier discharge to home.[18,23–25] Although there are studies that cite the use of buprenorphine in treatment of NAS, most of the literature discusses the effects of neonatal exposure to buprenorphine in utero in relation to development of NAS symptoms.[26,27] When in utero exposure occurs, infants may present with delayed signs and symptoms of NAS and require lower total opioid for treatment.[26,27]

In addition to a primary drug, such as morphine or methadone, some neonates require a secondary drug to control NAS symptoms. The 2 primary pharmacologic agents used for adjunctive therapy are phenobarbital and clonidine. A 2013 study by Surran and colleagues[28] describes a randomized prospective trial comparing phenobarbital and clonidine in efforts to reduce length of stay and treatment days with morphine. Although the group receiving phenobarbital was off morphine at a statistically significant earlier time, they were not medication-free and required home administration of phenobarbital for as long as 8 months. Infants receiving clonidine were on morphine for longer, but at the end of treatment they were drug-free.

Although tincture of opium is still used in some facilities for NAS treatment, there is concern due to the high alcohol content and toxic ingredients of the medication.[11] Unfortunately, a recently released evidence-based care sheet indicates that tincture of opium is the preferred first-line drug for symptomatic NAS.[29]

Table 2
Drugs used for treatment of neonatal abstinence syndrome

Drug	Dose	Advantages	Disadvantages	References Citing Use of This Drug
Primary Drugs				
Morphine[a]	0.05–0.2 mg/kg/dose q3–4 h Max dose 1.3 mg/kg/d	No alcohol Short half-life (9 h)	Sedation Apnea Constipation Frequent Dosing	Brown et al, [18] 2015 O'Brien et al, [20]2015 Stempniak, [21]2016 Liu et al, [22] 2011 Patrick et al, [23]2014 Young et al,[24] 2015
Methadone	0.05 –0.1/mg/kg/dose q 12 h Max dose 1 mg/kg/d	Long half-life (26 h) 12 hourly doses Associated with shorter hospitalization time	Longer duration of treatment even with shorter hospitalization Alcohol 8% Frequent follow-up needed	Brown et al, [18] 2015 Patrick et al, [23]2014 Young et al,[24] 2015 Gaalema et al, [26] 2012 Lee et al,[25] 2015
Buprenorphine	Dose 4–5 micrograms/kg/dose q8 h Max dose 60 micrograms/kg/day	Sublingual route Half-life (12 h) which allows levels to be monitored	Alcohol 30% which is almost as high as tincture of opium. Adjuvant medications required Limited amount of research available about effectiveness of drug.	Gaalema et al,[26] 2012 Lee et al,[25] 2015
Secondary Drugs				
Phenobarbital	Loading dose 16 mg/kg Maintenance dose 1–4 mg/kg/q12 h	Long half-life (45–100 h) Levels can be monitored	High treatment failure Interacts with other drugs Alcohol content is about 15% which is high for a secondary drug Sedation	Patrick et al, [23] 2014 Lee et al,[25] 2015 Surran et al,[28] 2013
Clonidine	Initial dose 0.5–1 microgram/kg followed by 0.5–1.25 micrograms/kg per dose q 4–6 h	Non-narcotic antagonist No sedation No alcohol Long half-life (44–72 h)	Hypotension Abrupt discontinuation may cause rapid rise of blood pressure and heart rate	Lee et al,[25] 2015 Surran et al,[28] 2013

[a] In earlier work diluted tincture of opium (DTO) was used in lieu of morphine but the tincture contained up to 45% alcohol. In most cases this has been replaced by oral morphine drops.

Data from [Dose] Kocherlakota P. Neonatal abstinence syndrome. Pediatrics 2014;134(2):e555.

Alternative Therapy

It is common to start treatment of opioid exposed infants with expectant management until the results of clinical assessments suggest the need for pharmacologic intervention; however, little attention has been paid to nonpharmacologic interventions. Alternative therapy may provide either full symptom relief or an adjunct to pharmacologic intervention and includes the use of acupuncture and other nontraditional treatment protocols for the relief of the symptoms of NAS. Two particular interventions are of note because there is sound research documenting effectiveness. One protocol comes from work in the United States the other is based on international research.

The first intervention is vibrotactile stimulation, where the researchers investigated the use of stochastic vibrotactile stimulation applied through a specially constructed mattress to 26 opioid exposed neonates (>37 weeks, 16/26 male subjects) for alternating cycles over a 6-hour to 8-hour treatment cycle.[30] All neonates in the study were already being maintained on drugs for treatment of symptomatic NAS and had been continuously hospitalized since birth. Results of the study were promising, with infants evidencing a 35% reduction in abnormal movements during stochastic vibrotactile stimulation on time. There was also a significant reduction in tachypnea and tachycardia and greater evidence of normal breathing patterns and heart rate significant at the $P<.03$ level.[30] Although this is a single-unit small study and as such not yet generalizable to larger populations of NAS infants, the study received competitive extramural funding from the National Institute on Drug Abuse (R01 DA042074–01 [EBS]) and the National Institutes of Health (NIDA R21DA035355 EBS), which means there was rigorous scientific scrutiny of the research design and methodology.

The other treatment included as alternative therapy for NAS is acupuncture. There is literature first described in 1971 by a German researcher Gunter Lange calling the outer rim of the ear the "vegetative rim" due to its close approximation to the acupuncture points located near the ear helix.[31] The Kurath-Koller and colleagues[31] study described was used without pharmacologic support for NAS and all infants were managed in the NICU. Because the study was conducted in Austria, with a low incidence of NAS, the investigators caution that findings should be replicated and that other studies use acupuncture as complementary rather than alternative care. Raith and colleagues[32] also report on the use of laser acupuncture as a complementary care with significant reduction in days of pharmacologic management with opioids for NAS infants.

Family Therapy

A growing area in the clinical management of NAS is the concept of family-based intervention for care. This strategy of intervention is directed around the concept that many of the pharmacologic interventions for NAS infants may be better positioned as attempts to create healthier families. To that end, efforts to withdraw mothers from opioids prior to delivery are among many family strategies in place. The availability and assessment of relative safety of less addictive drugs for maternal treatment means that many addictions providers have moved away from methadone to buprenorphine.[25,26]

With efforts to focus on the family, 2 particular interventions are important. The first is the role of maternal-infant bonding. The second and somewhat related intervention is the role of breastfeeding. In many of the original treatment protocols for NAS, the infant was maintained in the NICU and kept at a distance from the mother, even if the infant was not intrauterine growth retarded or otherwise compromised at birth. The clinical judgment was that any emerging signs of developing symptomatic NAS with increasing scores on assessments needed to be able to be observed, which needed to take place in the presence of trained staff. In many cases, the mothers were not trusted to care for their own infants due to their social history. Fortunately, attention in the addiction treatment community is focusing on the maternal-infant attachment relationship and it is this same relationship that also provides the most cost-effective NAS treatment.[33] But according to Knopf[33] and researchers at Yale New Haven Children's Hospital,

> *If you stay out of the NICU, standardize non-pharmacologic care and empower parents...you get a reduction in the percentage of infants treated with morphine from 98 percent to 14 percent, a reduction in average length of stay (ALOS) from 22.4 to 5.9 days and a decrease in costs from $44,824 to $10,289.*

The research team developed and standardized 8 interventions that aimed at reducing average length of stay of neonates with NAS and although pharmacologic agents were not withheld if needed, the focus was developing a health family unit. Breastfeeding was also encouraged unless there was a contraindication, such as HIV or illicit drug use.

Despite the successful family intervention program reported by Knopf, researchers do not regularly consider breastfeeding status a variable to include in data collection in NAS research. Anderson[34] in a letter to the editor raised the question about whether Young and colleagues[24] considered breastfeeding among the confounding variable in their chart review. The editor responded that the authors had not considered collecting breastfeeding data.

DISEASE COMPLICATIONS

Complications of NAS during the immediate newborn period are generally limited to the complications of intrauterine growth retardation, prematurity, or complications related to withdrawal from the opioids.[11] Because these substances cross the placenta, availability terminates with birth and symptoms of withdrawal can occur across a spectrum.[35]

Due to the effects of the opioids on the developing brain, there can be short-term and long-term effects on neurodevelopment. Recent literature also has identified effects on brain size and weight and on the development of numerous neurotransmitters.[22]

TECHNIQUES

Techniques that are applicable to the care of NAS infants include comprehensive maternal and neonatal assessment, including specialized NAS scoring, counseling of mothers, and other members of the household regarding illicit substance abuse; support in nonpharmacologic interventions; development of effective communication techniques between all members of the care team; support of breastfeeding if it is not contraindicated; and recognition that the need to use pharmacologic treatment does not represent maternal failure at efforts to stay clean of opioids.

EVIDENCE

Evidence of each of the recommended interventions has been provided throughout the article. There are 2 sets of evidence-based practice guidelines, however, that may help readers decipher the sources for current nursing practice recommendations. The first, described by Schub and Karakashian,[29] is an Evidence-Based Care Sheet on

Neonatal Abstinence Syndrome, published by Cinahl Information Systems, a division of EBSCO Information Services. The sheet provides bulleted information with references for each bullet. References are coded based on the type of information sources, for example, published guidelines by a professional association, randomized controlled trial, or published funded report.

The second is a research article by Boucher[36] that searched PubMed, Ovid MEDLINE, Embase, and CINAHL databases for primary studies on rooming-in care and acupuncture as adjunctive treatments for NAS. The article reviewed 8 evidence-based practice studies. Unlike the first evidence-based care sheet, this article focuses on the nonpharmacologic interventions where nursing can make a real difference in family outcomes.

CONTROVERSIES

Current controversies in the care and treatment of prenatal opioid use and NAS can be categorized as (1) those that relate to the handling of women who are addicted either to opioids or street drugs and whether they should be treated in the criminal system or in the drug treatment system; (2) whether naltrexone (Vivitrol), an untested drug in pregnancy, should be mandated for administration to pregnant women with a history of opioid use; and (3) what role a substance using mother should play in the care and management of her newborn child if that addiction is a form of child abuse. These controversies lead to several policy decisions at a time when health care costs and outcomes are under serious scrutiny.

The first controversial issue defines the paradigm of how NAS is addressed—as a result of a criminal offense or as a treatable disease. This shifting paradigm has allowed novel approaches to newborn treatment with more cost effective care models. An article by Gaspari,[37] however, describes the case of Mallory Loyola, who gave birth to a baby girl who tested positive for methamphetamine in 2014 in Tennessee. She was charged on July 8, 2014, for simple assault under Tennessee's statute that criminalized drug use in pregnancy. Although the charges were later dropped in 2015 after Loyola completed a drug rehabilitation program and stayed "drug free" for 6 months, she will not be the last pregnant women charged with a criminal offense for addicting her fetus while in utero. Tennessee took the desperate action of criminalizing the consumption of maternal drugs during pregnancy due to the rapid increase in opioid use in the state and in NAS. Although the goal is to determine if criminal consequences of substance use in pregnancy curb behavior, the law is scheduled to sunset in 2 years after it is evaluated. Although Tennessee has gone the criminal route, 18 other states consider it a civil issue falling under the child welfare system and 3 states can commit a mother to inpatient treatment. Alabama and South Carolina have upheld convictions for criminal child abuse in mothers who are substance abusers despite not having a criminal statute.[37]

Just as whether substance abuse in pregnant women is treated as a criminal offense, the second area of controversy is whether pregnant women should be allowed to control the medications they are forced to take. Two reports from the substance abuse literature discuss draft recommendations from the Substance Abuse and Mental Health Services Administration on prenatal opioid exposure and development of NAS.[38,39] In these draft recommendations, which are now out for public comment, naltrexone (Vivitrol) is an agonist agent given to women during pregnancy to decrease or eliminate their opioid addiction. Unfortunately, naltrexone is a category C drug, which means there is no information on the established safety of this drug in pregnancy.

The final controversy related to an abusing mother's role in the care of her newborn is discussed previously. This is an area where nurses have an opportunity to make significant impact on decisions that improve care and improve quality of outcomes for their patients. It is interesting that the nursing perspective is absent from the editorial by Chasnoff and Gardner,[40] purporting to espouse the policy perspective on NAS without discussing the need to support cost-effective alternative care, which may include alternative and complementary care and breast-feeding if not contraindicated by active drug use or HIV.

PROGNOSIS

Infants who have been exposed to opioids prenatally may have cognitive delays and suffer anxiety, aggression, and disruptive or inattentive behaviors later in life.[13] Although there have been improvements in care options and treatment modalities, NAS is still a potentially serious disorder at the time of birth and long-term due to the brain abnormalities present initially and those along with neurodevelopmental findings that develop over time, some of which are still being identified.

SUMMARY

The challenge for nurses remains to equip families with the skills to make informed decisions about substance use. Nurses also become engaged in facilitating mothers in becoming active participants in their infant's care. Most importantly, nurses help mothers and families develop attachments that in the past might have been difficult due to the barriers society put in place within the systems of care.

REFERENCES

1. World Drug Report 2017. World Drug Report. 2017. https://doi.org/10.18356/c595e10f-en. Available at: www.undoc.org/wdr2017/en/exsum.html. Accessed December 12, 2017.
2. National Institute on Drug Abuse (NIDA). National Institutes of Health. US Department of Health and Human Services. Advancing addiction science. Dramatic increase in maternal opioid use and Neonatal Abstinence Syndrome. 2015. Available at: http://www.drugabuse.gov/related topics-statistics/infographics/dramatic increase in maternal opioid-use-neonatal abstinence-syndrome. Accessed December 7, 2017.
3. Mcqueen K, Murphy-Oikonen J. Neonatal abstinence syndrome. N Engl J Med 2016;375(25):2468–79.
4. Hudak ML, Tan RC. Committee on drugs; committee on fetus and newborn; American Academy of Pediatrics. Neonatal drug withdrawal. Pediatrics 2012; 129(2):e540–60.
5. Substance Abuse and Mental Health Services Administration. Results from the 2013 national survey on drug use and health: summary of national findings, NSDUH. Series 4-48. HHS Publication No (SMA) 14-486 3. Rockville (MD): Substance Abuse and Mental Health Services Administration; 2014.
6. Shannon J, Blythe S, Peters K. Neonatal abstinence syndrome and the attachment relationship. Aust Nurs Midwifery J 2016;24(6):42. Available from: Academic Search Complete, Ipswich, MA. Available at: https://europepmc.org/abstract/MED/29251895. Accessed December 18, 2017.

7. Weiss AJ, Elixhauser A, Barrett ML, et al. Opioid-related inpatient stays and emergency department visits by state.2009-2014. HCUP statistical brief #219. 1-16.
8. Ko JV, Patrick SW, Tong VT, et al. Incidence of neonatal abstinence Syndrome-28 states 1999-2014. MMWR Morb Mortal Wkly Rep 2016;65:799–802.
9. Tolia VN, Patrick SW, Bennett MW, et al. Increasing incidence of the neonatal abstinence syndrome in US neonatal ICUs. N Engl J Med 2015;372(22):2118–26.
10. Osborn DA, Jeffery HE, Cole MJ. Opiate treatment for opiate withdrawal in newborn infants. Cochrane Database Syst Rev 2010;(10):CD002059. Available at: http://pqcnc-documents.s3.amazonaws.com/nas/nasprework/general/PQCNCNASCochranDatabase.pdf. Accessed December 18, 2017.
11. Kocherlakota P. Neonatal abstinence syndrome. Pediatrics 2014;134(2):e547–61.
12. Reddy UM, Davis Ren Z, Green MF. Opioid use in pregnancy, neonatal abstinence syndrome, and childhood outcomes: executive summary of a joint workshop by the Eunice Kennedy Shriver National Institute of Child Health and Human Development, American College of Obstetricians and Gynecologists, American Academy of Pediatrics, Society for Maternal-Fetal Medicine, Centers for Disease Control and Prevention, and the March of Dimes Foundation. Obstet Gynecol 2017;130(1):10–28.
13. Jensen CL. Improving outcomes for infants with NAS. The Clinical Advisor: 2014; 85–92. Available at: www.ClinicalAdvisor.com. Accessed December 7, 2017.
14. Murphy-Oikonen J, Montelpare WJ, Bertoldo L, et al. The impact of a clinical practice guideline on infants with neonatal abstinence syndrome. Br J Midwifery 2012;20(7):493–501.
15. Orlando S. An overview of clinical tools used to assess neonatal abstinence syndrome. J Perinat Neonatal Nurs 2014;28(3):212–9.
16. Rosen M. Shaky start. Sci News 2017;191(11):16–20.
17. Nayeri F, Ebrahim B, Shariat M, et al. Treating neonatal abstinence syndrome from clinical perspectives. Iran J Pediatr 2017;27(4):1–4.
18. Brown MS, Hayes MJ, Thornton LM. Methadone versus morphine for treatment of neonatal abstinence syndrome: a prospective randomized clinical trial. J Perinatol 2015;35:278–83.
19. Hudak ML, Tan RC. Clinical report: Neonatal drug withdrawal. AAP The Committee on Drugs and The Committee on Fetus and Newborn. https://doi.org/10.1542/peds.2011-321. Available at: www.pediatrics.org/cgi/doi/10.1542/peds.2011-3212. http://pediatrics.aappublications.org/content/pediatrics/129/2/e540.full.pdf. Accessed December 17, 2017.
20. O'Brien JE, Dumas H, Leslie D. Neonatal abstinence outcomes in post-acute care: a brief report. J Pediatr Rehabil Med 2015;8:157–60.
21. Stempniak M. Costly condition. Hospitals try new approaches to treating opioid-dependent babies. Hosp Health Netw 2016;90(6):14. Available from: CINAHL Complete, Ipswich, MA. Available at: http://proxy.cc.uic.edu/login?url=http://search.ebscohost.com/login.aspx?direct=true&db=hch&AN=116407279. Accessed December 17, 2017.
22. Liu A, Björkman T, Stewart C, et al. Pharmacological treatment of neonatal opiate withdrawal: between the devil and the deep blue sea. Int J Pediatr 2011;2011: 1–5. Available from: Academic Search Complete, Ipswich, MA. Available at: http://proxy.cc.uic.edu/login?url=http://search.ebscohost.com/login.aspx?direct=true&db=a9h&AN=70785199. Accessed December 20, 2017.
23. Patrick S, Kaplan H, Passarella M, et al. Variation in treatment of neonatal abstinence syndrome in US Children's Hospitals, 2004-2011. J Perinatol 2014;34(11):867–72.

CINAHL Complete, Ipswich, MA. Available at: http://proxy.cc.uic.edu/login?url=http://search.ebscohost.com/login.aspx?direct=true&db=hch&AN=99626913. Accessed December 17, 2017.

24. Young M, Hager S, Spurlock D. Retrospective chart review comparing morphine and methadone in neonates treated for neonatal abstinence syndrome. Am J Health Syst Pharm 2015;72:S162–7. CINAHL Complete, Ipswich, MA. Available at: http://proxy.cc.uic.edu/login?url=search.ebscohost.com/login.aspx?direct=true&db=a9h&AN=111323244. Accessed December 17, 2017.
25. Lee J, Hulman S, Musci M, et al. Neonatal abstinence syndrome: influence of a combined inpatient/outpatient methadone treatment regimen on the average length of stay of a medicaid NICU population. Popul Health Manag 2015;18(5):392–7. CINAHL Complete, Ipswich, MA. Available at: http://proxy.cc.uic.edu/login?url=http://search.ebscohost.com/login.aspx?direct=true&db=rzh&AN=109467293. Accessed December 18, 2017.
26. Gaalema D, Scott T, Jones H, et al. Differences in the profile of neonatal abstinence syndrome signs in methadone- versus buprenorphine-exposed neonates. Addiction 2012; 107:53–62. CINAHL Complete, Ipswich, MA. Available at: http://proxy.cc.uic.edu/login?url=http://search.ebscohost.com/login.aspx?direct=true&db=a9h&AN=82891934. Accessed December 17, 2017.
27. Decker T, Kulick M, Lyng A, et al. Assessment and treatment of neonatal abstinence syndrome: a review of the literature. counselor. The Magazine For Addiction Professionals [serial online] 2017;18(6):28–34. Available from: CINAHL Complete, Ipswich, MA. Accessed December 19, 2017.
28. Surran B, Visintainer P, Chamberlain S, et al. Efficacy of clonidine versus phenobarbital in reducing neonatal morphine sulfate therapy days for neonatal abstinence syndrome. A prospective randomized clinical trial. J Perinatol 2013; 33(12):954–9. Available from: CINAHL Complete, Ipswich, MA. Available at: http://proxy.cc.uic.edu/login?url=http://search.ebscohost.com/login.aspx?direct=true&db=hch&AN=92579222. Accessed December 18, 2017.
29. Schub T, Karakashian A. Neonatal abstinence syndrome. CINAHL Nursing Guide [serial online]. 2017. CINAHL Complete, Ipswich, MA. Available at: http://proxy.cc.uic.edu/login?url=http://search.ebscohost.com/login.aspx?direct=true&db=rzh&AN=T701827. Accessed December 19, 2017.
30. Zuzarte I, Indic P, Barton B, et al. Vibrotactile stimulation: a non-pharmacological intervention for opioid-exposed newborns. PLoS One 2017;12(4):e0175981.
31. Kurath-Koller S, Pansy J, Mileder L, et al. Active somatic and psychic ear acupuncture points in newborn infants with neonatal abstinence syndrome. J Altern Complement Med 2016;22(10):788–93. Available from: Academic Search Complete, Ipswich, MA. Accessed December 19, 2017.
32. Raith W, Schmblzer G, Urlesberger B, et al. Laser acupuncture for neonatal abstinence syndrome: a randomized controlled trial. Pediatrics 2015;136(5):876–84. Academic Search Complete, Ipswich, MA. Available at: http://pediatrics.aappublications.org.proxy.cc.uic.edu/content/136/5/876. Accessed December 19, 2017.
33. Knopf A. Best - and least costly - treatment for NAS is mother-infant bond. Alcoholism & Drug Abuse Weekly [serial online] 2017;29(23):4–6. Academic Search Complete, Ipswich, MA. Available at: http://proxy.cc.uic.edu/login?url=http://search.ebscohost.com/login.aspx?direct=true&db=hxh&AN=123543373. Accessed December 19, 2017.
34. Anderson P. Effect of breastfeeding on neonatal abstinence syndrome. Am J Health Syst Pharm 2016;73(12):864. Academic Search Complete, Ipswich, MA.

Available at: http://proxy.cc.uic.edu/login?url=http://search.ebscohost.com/login.aspx?direct=true&db=hch&AN=115889835. Accessed December 19, 2017.
35. Patrick SW, Schiff DM, AAP Committee on Substance Use and Prevention. A public health response to opioid use in pregnancy. Pediatrics 2017;139(3):e2016407.
36. Boucher AM. Non-opioid management of neonatal abstinence syndrome. Adv Neonatal Care 2017;17(2):84–90.
37. Gaspari A. Inheriting your mother's eyes, hair, and drug addiction: protecting the drug-exposed newborn by criminalizing pregnant drug use. Fam Court Rev 2016; 54(1):96–111.
38. Hunt JM. Naltrexone during pregnancy being considered due to prenatal opioid exposure. Brown University Child & Adolescent Psychopharmacology Update [serial online] 2017;19(3):1–3. Available at: http://proxy.cc.uic.edu/login?url=http://search.ebscohost.com/login.aspx?direct=true&db=a9h&AN=121443609. Accessed December 20, 2017.
39. Knopf A. SAMHSA draft report on NAS discusses Vivitrol during pregnancy. Alcoholism & Drug Abuse Weekly [serial online] 2017;29(6):1–4. Academic Search Complete, Ipswich, MA. Available at: Available at: http://proxy.cc.uic.edu/login?url=http://search.ebscohost.com/login.aspx?direct=true&db=a9h&AN=121118034. Accessed December 20, 2017.
40. Chasnoff I, Gardner S. Neonatal abstinence syndrome: a policy perspective. J Perinatol 2015;35(8):539–41. Available from: Academic Search Complete, Ipswich, MA. Accessed December 20, 2017.

Neonatal Transport

Current Trends and Practices

Beth C. Diehl, DNP, NNP-BC, CCRN, LNCC*

KEYWORDS

• Neonatal • Transport • Team • Regionalization • Training • Accreditation

KEY POINTS

- Program accreditation-transport programs are beginning to embrace the concept of accreditation to assure competency and compliance with transport standards and explore avenues for accreditation.
- Transport team training simulation-based training that addresses clinical competence for low-volume high-risk procedures in conjunction with leadership and communication skills minimizes adverse event occurrences.
- The ability to provide active versus passive cooling for transported neonates with HIE minimizes the occurrence of overcooling and achieves target zone temperatures more readily.
- Technological advances now allow for high-frequency ventilation to be utilized in the transport environment, which can meet the respiratory needs of the most critically ill neonates.
- The measurement of outcomes related to effectiveness, safety, efficiency, family/patient centeredness, and timeliness of the high-risk transport environment is essential for quality care.

INTRODUCTION AND THE NECESSITY AND PROCESS OF NEONATAL TRANSPORT

The transport of newborns has been a necessity for many decades when it became clinically apparent that not all hospitals could provide the level of care required by a premature or critically ill neonate. Derived from the Latin words of portare, meaning to carry and trans, meaning across, the transportation of neonates at risk for morbidities and mortality took hold.[1] This realization of the need existed even before the advent of modern-day neonatal intensive care units (NICUs). Despite best efforts to arrange for maternal antenatal transfer when dictated by clinical status, it is not always feasible from a logistical or safety standpoint. Hence, there will inevitably be neonates

Disclosure: The author has nothing to disclose.
Maryland Regional Neonatal Transport Program, Johns Hopkins Hospital, Charlotte Bloomberg Children's Center, Room 8547, 1800 Orleans Street, Baltimore, MD 21287, USA
* Corresponding author. 22 Tigreff Court, Baltimore, MD 21234-1444.
E-mail address: Bdiehls1@jhmi.edu

Crit Care Nurs Clin N Am 30 (2018) 597–606
https://doi.org/10.1016/j.cnc.2018.07.012
ccnursing.theclinics.com

who will require an emergent or semiemergent transfer during their hospital course after birth from a lower to a higher level of neonatal care.

Many decades have passed since the late 1930s to 1940s and with it the establishment of regionalized neonatal care. However, neonatal transport remains an essential and ever evolving subspecialty and a true outgrowth of regionalization. The concept of regionalization as the model of distribution of perinatal health care is the linking of hospitals in a coordinated system of communication, learning, and response.[2] Organized neonatal transport systems were initially designed and implemented by US public health programs.[1] External forces in recent decades such as those related to regulatory policy, financial affiliations, population density and marketing patterns have added a new layer of complexity and challenge for existing and newly formed perinatal networks and thus the world of neonatal transport.

Neonatal transport rapidly became an important element in the perinatal care model. To this day, the transport environment remains dynamic and complex. Transporting a neonate to a place of definitive treatment where the appropriate resources and expertise are available is embedded in the concepts of equitable access to necessary health care facilities.[3] There exist hospitals with delivery services but without a NICU. Even among hospitals that house a NICU, there are varying levels of capacity for delivering neonatal care.[4] The establishment and preservation of a perinatal network provides a safeguard for all mothers and neonates who require differing levels of clinical care and follow-up.

Neonatal patients have needs that exist as a consequence of prematurity, respiratory insufficiency, acute infection, genetic conditions, and congenital anomalies of anatomy and physiology, or as a result of unexpected perinatal events. The safe and secure transport of infants in critical or unstable condition requires highly dependable interprofessional transport teams. These teams should be competently trained with the necessary equipment and supplies to provide care in inexperienced, often chaotic, and resource-limited environments.[5]

The coordination of the transport of neonates, some from significant geographic distances, is customarily initiated with a call to a level 3 or 4 neonatal center. With the exchange of information regarding current clinical status, a determination of the urgency for transport, facility placement selection depending on the individual perinatal network, and the exact mode of transport, decisions are then made for the transport to be executed. Once dispatched from the base hospital and upon the arrival at the referral facility, the transport team has the responsibility of assessment and clinical stabilization of the neonate. This process includes the handoff of information from the referral physician, nurse, and possibly respiratory therapist, as well as an update and bedside visit to the mother and any other family members present prior to departure. The transport team will then continue to provide intensive care during transport, whether it is by fixed-wing or rotor-winged aircraft or ambulance. Upon arrival at the receiving NICU, the transport team is responsible for informing the accepting medical and nursing team of any clinical or logistical events that transpired during transit, as well as providing a comprehensive and safe handoff of care.

HISTORY/CURRENT STATISTICS

In the United States, there are 68,979 neonates transported annually or approximately 188 transports undertaken daily.[6] Admission rates to NICUs have been increasing related to overall population growth in the United States. Prior to the twentieth century, most births occurred in the home, with neonatal morbidity or mortality a relatively common occurrence given the novel status of neonatal medicine at that time.[1,2] The fundamental desire to provide for the care of premature and critically ill neonates in the early nineteenth century prompted the manufacture of a portable incubator in the city of Chicago for neonatal transport. Interestingly, the Departments of Health in Chicago and New York City were among the first to have dedicated transport teams in the late 1940s.[1,2] Perhaps it was the urbanization of these areas that impelled this transport initiative. Whatever the circumstance or driving force, the first organized transportation program was enacted in 1948 by the New York Department of Health. The program possessed many tenets of current day neonatal transport programs: specially trained nurses available 24 hours a day, 7 days a week; a dedicated vehicle; an individual in charge of call recordings; and required equipment. Between the years of 1948 to 1950, 1209 neonates were transported in the New York geographic region, 194 of those neonates with birth weights under 1000 g and considered in the extremely low birth weight category and within the highest risk strata.[1] These initial efforts of neonatal transport set the stage for further development in equipment capabilities but also allowed for a critical appraisal of processes. This degree of appraisal resulted in the development of protocols and care safeguards for the neonate and the individual members of the transport team.

Subsequently, in the 1960s and 1970s, hospital-based neonatal transport teams continued to arise out of necessity using resources and clinicians from tertiary hospitals' neonatal units to retrieve infants. This practice was based on the inherent principle that these units were in the most optimal position to provide services based on education, knowledge, and experience regarding the care of premature and critically ill neonates.[2,5] As the regionalization of neonatal care became commonplace and transport programs proliferated and expanded, there was evidence of positive outcomes related to morbidity and mortality. According to the US Centers for Disease Control and Prevention, infant mortality declined by an average of 4.5% per year from 1965 to 1981.[1] Although this statistic encompasses evolving care protocols and durable medical equipment advances, it is reasonable to conclude that regionalization and the expedient and safe transport of ill neonates by trained transport teams contributed to the reduction of infant mortality rates.

In the early 1990s, leaders in the field of neonatal medicine and nursing met at a consensus-building conference to outline recommendations to define the minimum requirements for safe and effective transport of neonates. In 1990, the American Academy of Pediatrics (AAP) established the Section on Transport Medicine, and in 1993, the AAP published the initial Guidelines for Air and Ground Transportation of Neonatal and Pediatric Patients. The guidelines are updated periodically and serve to assist clinicians and transport and hospital administrators in terms of care protocols, legal/ethical issues, family considerations, documentation, and data collection.[1]

Neonatal transport teams now exist in countries around the globe in both industrialized and developing nations, with the ultimate goal of achieving a perinatal infrastructure that supports all neonates at risk for potential morbidity or mortality.[7,8] Efforts continue within the neonatal community through education, evidence-based research, and emerging technologies to provide the most optimally educated team. In addition, there are ongoing initiatives to develop equipment that is ergonomically appropriate and sufficiently compact for transport ambulances and aircraft.

The AAP issued a policy statement in 2012 that classified treatment centers offering neonatal care into 4 levels. This was an update from a previous designation that provided for 3 levels of neonatal care, with subdivisions within levels 2 and 3. This most recent version provided clarity to regional networks but also to the lay public. Consumer interest in care capabilities has become commonplace with the availability of the Internet and a heightened awareness related to outcomes and services. The delineation of the levels into 4 categories reflected overall advances in neonatal medicine and nursing and the quantity of subspecialists needed to care for the most complex and challenging neonate.[9] **Box 1** delineates the 4 levels of care.

ACCREDITATION REQUIREMENTS

Regulations governing transport have been sparse historically but continue to evolve, and when enacted, impact neonatal transport delivery on a national and/or state level. Risks need to be considered and managed effectively to ensure the safety of all involved. All neonatal team members need to be knowledgeable of alterations in neonatal physiology that occur during ambulance or helicopter transport of a critically ill neonate related to weather conditions, temperature extremes, equipment issues, and vehicle mishaps.[10] Although many transport programs are not currently accredited, there is movement toward accreditation in the transport environment. To assure that competency and compliance with transport standards of care, 5 agencies exist that provides regulatory oversight:

1. Commission on Accreditation of Medical Transport Systems (CAMTS, www.camts.org) is an organization of nonprofit organizations dedicated to improving the quality and safety of medical transport services. The commission offers a program of voluntary evaluation of compliance with accreditation standards demonstrating the ability to deliver service of a specific quality with the 2 highest priorities of a transport service being patient care and safety of the transport environment. Originally developed and published in 1991 and revised every 2 to 3 years, the accreditation standards address issues of patient care and safety in fixed- and rotary-wing aircraft, as well as ground interfacility ambulance teams providing critical care transports. Each standard is supported by measurable criteria to measure a program's level of quality.[11]
2. The Commission on Accreditation of Ambulance Services (CASS, www.cass.org) was established to encourage and promote quality patient care in America's medical transportation system. CAAS is an independent commission that established a comprehensive series of standards for the ambulance service industry. CAAS accreditation signifies that the service has met the gold standard determined by the ambulance industry to be essential in a modern emergency medical services

Box 1
Perinatal level of care designations

Level 1: Well newborn nurseries providing basic level care to neonates who are low risk and have capabilities for neonatal resuscitation

Level 2: Care reserved for stable or moderately ill newborn infants born at >32 weeks' gestation or birth weights >1500 g with problems that are expected to resolve rapidly and who would not be anticipated to require subspecialty level services on an urgent basis

Level 3: Care in NICUs having continuously available personnel (neonatologists, neonatal nurses, respiratory therapists) and equipment to provide life support for as long as necessary. These centers have pediatric subspecialists and pediatric surgery services.

Level 4: These consist of level 3 care with additional capabilities and experience in the care of the most complex and critically ill newborn infants.

Data from Committee on Fetus and Newborn. Levels of neonatal care. Pediatrics 2012;13(3):587–97.

provider. The CAAS standards are designed to increase operational efficiency and clinical quality, while decreasing risk and liability to the organization. The process includes a comprehensive self-assessment and an independent external review of the emergency medical services organization.[12]

3. The National Alliance of Medical Transport Applications (NAAMTA, www.naamta.com) is the new accreditation standard bearer for the medical transport industry, offering procedures that include guidelines for developing a quality management system focusing on transport safety, patient care, and continuous improvement. Since its inception in 2009, NAAMTA has identified key best practices to improve the standard of performance among medical transport systems at the global level.[13]
4. Since 1994, the Joint Commission International (JCI, www.jointcommissioninternational.org) has been the world's largest health care accreditor. The JCI standards address all aspects of emergency and nonemergency transport of patients that apply to public and community-based medical transport organizations associated with hospitals.[14]
5. The European Aero-Medical Institute (EURAMI, www.eurami.org) promotes high-quality aeromedical transfers throughout Europe and the world via fixed-wing or rotor aircrafts through research, training, and accreditation in the field of aeromedical transfers.[15]

The pathway to accreditation for each organization or agency varies in terms of the application process, time line and fees, geographic jurisdiction, and renewal requirements. Neonatal transport programs will need to carefully examine the best pathway to accreditation from an organizational perspective if there is a desire to achieve accreditation status. Statistics vary as to the number of programs currently accredited in the United States. As such, accreditation will continue to be an evolving issue for transport programs given the cost, degree of institutional support available, preparation time needed for an accreditation visit, and cost/benefit ratio of possessing an accredited team. More research is needed to substantiate any direct link between the existence of accreditation and improved outcomes in the transport arena.

SIMULATION-BASED TRAINING/SKILLS ASSESSMENT

As neonatal transport became a professionally acknowledged subspecialty, the most effective manner in which to train the transport team personnel was debated among educators and clinicians. Given that transport team composition varies in the United States and each provider is functioning within his or her individual scope of practice, the educational process is challenging. In 2011, Karlsen completed a national survey of neonatal transport teams in the United States and found that 44.3% of neonatal transports are completed by a nurse-respiratory therapist team. A nurse-nurse team is the second most commonly utilized team, servicing approximately 11.3% of transports. Interestingly, the neonatal nurse practitioner-nurse team is utilized for only 4.7% of neonatal transports in the United States.[6] The other important factor regarding training is the ability of the providers to function as a team, as well as individuals to foster clear communication, and embrace the designated leadership role with the ultimate goal of avoiding adverse events. This is particularly difficult within a nondedicated team structure when personnel can be intermittently and randomly sourced for transport calls.

Generally, didactic content, observation, and performance of procedures are commonly employed methods for transport team training. However, establishing competence for low-volume, high-risk procedures remains problematic (eg, needle aspiration of pneumothorax or endotracheal intubation). In addition, team communication and leadership were found to be factors in sentinel events. Specifically, in 2004, the Joint Commission on Accreditation of Healthcare Organizations (JCAHO) published a sentinel event alert after evaluating 109 transport-related cases. Root cause analysis determined that 72% of cases had miscommunication and poor team work factors; 47% involved questions of staff competency, and 40% related to the lack of appropriate training.[16] Action was required on a nationwide level to address these deficiencies. Simulation training, combined with team leadership, was shown to be as effective for skill development as traditional methods.

Simulation-based education has become the norm not only for unit-based training, but certainly for the training of transport team personnel. It can be done simply via the creation and execution of case based scenarios in a low technology environment or in the presence of simulation centers and high-fidelity equipment that offers real-time feedback to the learner. Specifically, the concepts of psychological fidelity, which approximates the feel or realism of a situation, and physical fidelity, which is a replication of the physical attributes of the newborn or task or procedure being simulated are important elements to consider when training transport teams.[17] Resources vary widely between programs, both nationally and internationally, but the context of any training should include components of simulation for educational impact and to achieve high-level team and individual performance.

EVOLVING TRANSPORT THERAPIES/ACTIVE COOLING FOR NEUROPROTECTIVE HYPOTHERMIA

Perinatal hypoxic ischemic encephalopathy (HIE) can lead to severe neurodevelopmental outcome and death. In the early to mid-2000s, studies were conducted to evaluate the neuroprotective efficacy of hypothermia for the treatment of HIE. The studies involved 2 types of therapies: whole-body cooling or selective head cooling.[18] As the studies progressed and positive outcomes were demonstrated for neonates undergoing neuroprotective hypothermia, this therapy became standard of care. However, the time frames surrounding the cooling protocols became an issue for neonatal transport teams as well as the referral and accepting high-level regional NICUs; the neonate must be placed on active cooling via a cooling blanket system within 6 hours of birth to prevent the reperfusion injury associated with HIE.[19] Therapeutic hypothermia is performed in level 3 and 4 NICUs related to the need for specialized equipment, pediatric neurology involvement, and ongoing brain imaging and electrical monitoring. These neonates require subspecialty support services that are not a part of level 1 or level 2 nursery care capabilities.

HIE or neonatal encephalopathy (NE) can be the result of shoulder dystocia, cord prolapse, placental abruption, uterine rupture, or unintended birth trauma. These complications can occur in any level nursery and often are unanticipated at the time of delivery. Accordingly, once the determination of the need for neuroprotective hypothermia is determined after consult with the tertiary or quaternary care NICU, neonates need to be expediently transported to the higher level of care. Initially, the only option for referral hospital staff and transport team providers was to initiate passive cooling by terminating the external heat source and allowing the neonate to passively cool until the commonly accepted goal temp of 33.5° Celsius was reached.

Depending on the geographic distance between the facilities and the mode of transport, there could be significant fluctuation in the neonates' body temperature. The potential exists for the neonate to be overly cooled with a temperature below 33.5° C or goal treatment temperature not able to be reached prior to arrival at the referral center.

This is because of transit times, weather conditions, and other factors such as frequency of temperature monitoring. These fluctuating body temperatures prior to the neonate being placed on active cooling within 6 hours of age do not provide optimal therapy for neuroprotection.[20]

Within a few years of the institution of passive cooling, commercial products have become available to provide active cooling during transport. The Techotherm is one such active cooling product (http://www.maxtec.com/product/other/tecothermneo/). This unit has a fluid-filled blanket connected to a cooling unit with biofeedback via internal temperature probe. Studies have examined outcomes related to those neonates who were passively cooled versus actively cooled. Stafford and colleagues in 2014,[18] comparing a group of neonates passively versus actively cooled in transport found that there was greater variability in temperatures of the passively cooled group. A greater number of actively cooled patients arrived at the higher-level NICU within the goal temperature range than those passively cooled (79% vs 29% respectively). Accordingly, they found that active cooling was a significant independent predictor for arriving within the goal temperature range and recommended that active servo-controlled therapeutic hypothermia be used.

EVOLVING TRANSPORT THERAPIES/HIGH-FREQUENCY VENTILATION

High-frequency ventilation (HFV) has been integrated into neonatal care for essentially 2 plus decades. The use of HFV in the transport environment was limited until commercially manufactured transport ventilators became available. For clinical situations such as respiratory failure, significant air leak syndrome, and failure of conventional mechanical ventilation (CMV), the use of HFV can facilitate a more optimal transport for the neonate.[21] This is the case if neonates in level 3 centers require lateral transfer for subspecialty care currently being managed with HFV. Without HFV capability, the neonates would have to be transitioned back to CMV, potentially leading to clinical instability or decompensation during transit. Literature regarding the use of HFV in transport is sparse. Honey and colleagues[22] utilized the Duotron ventilator for 134 neonates transported in the Intermountain West region of the United States (Utah, Wyoming, Idaho, Montana, Arizona, Nevada, and Colorado). Most neonates 96% (n = 128) were successfully transported. Oxygen requirements were tracked before and after transport, as well as blood gas data. Inspired oxygen requirements remained unchanged or improved in most patients along with ventilation and acid-base balance.

Another HFV commercially available is the TXP, which is a pneumatically powered, pressure-limited, time-cycled, and high-frequency flow interrupter (https://int-bio.com/blog/intbio-products/high-frequency-ventilator/). It consists of the ventilator unit, phasitron, and circuit. The vent allows for carbon dioxide removal and oxygen diffusion. The phasitron portion is a mechanical interface that precisely delivers breaths to selected pressures and allows for oscillatory equilibrium. The ventilator circuit is open to ambient air, so the risk for barotrauma is minimal. However, the TXP does not have an active expiratory phase; rather this phase is passive. The TXP is portable and transport approved. Parameters for amplitude, high frequency rate, inspired oxygen concentration, and mean airway pressure (PAW) are set by the operator and are adjusted based on blood gas values, oxygen saturation levels, and clinical examination.

Although the TXP or any other HFV in transport can optimize patient care, the learning curve for transport personnel is significant. Education must be provided in both didactic and simulation format for a successful transition. Transport team leaders, nurse practitioners, and respiratory therapists must have full command of the capabilities of the device and be able to adapt quickly to environmental and clinical changes during transport. These include the difficulty in assessing chest wiggle with road vibration, avoidance of breaking the circuit for isolette loading and unloading events, and power disruptions that occur with the switch from battery to wall power.[22] In addition, ambulances and/or aircraft depending on the transport mode must have sufficient on-board oxygen and medical air to meet the gas consumption required by the device, especially on long distance ground transports. This is an area of clinical practice that requires further research to determine appropriate care algorithms, educational pathways, and adaptation to the transport environment as well as outcome data.

QUALITY METRICS

Neonatal transport is recognized as a high-risk activity with considerable threat of adverse events because of its inherent dynamic nature. Committing the proper resources and personnel in conjunction with tracking outcome metrics cannot be overemphasized. Ratnavel indicates that national bench marking as an evaluative component is essential to follow trends in patient acuity and measures the ability to comply with predesignated service standards.[3] Despite the sheer number of neonates transported nationally and internationally on a daily basis, practice variations remain that may result in suboptimal outcomes. Accordingly, the AAP, CAMTS, and the Air Medical Physician Association published operational and clinical care recommendations. Schwartz and colleagues[23] crafted a list of metrics rated as "very important" with the subcategories of effectiveness, safety, efficiency, family/patient centeredness, and timeliness. These metrics were organized by Institute of Medicine Quality Domains. The final quality metrics were stratified by weighted rank. See **Box 2** for all metrics that met the criteria as being very important with a 70% consensus.

These metrics have the ability for neonatal transport teams to benchmark performance and guide quality improvement efforts. These efforts have been similarly adopted on an international level and applied to adverse event tracking. Van den Berg and

Box 2
Quality metrics for neonatal transport

- Unplanned dislodgement of therapeutic devises
- Verification of tracheal tube placement
- Average mobilization time of the transport team
- First attempt tracheal tube placement
- Rate of transport-related injuries
- Rate of medication administration errors
- Rate of patient medical equipment failure during transport
- Rate of cardiopulmonary resuscitation performed during transport
- Rate of serious reportable events
- Unintended neonatal hypothermia upon arrival to destination
- Rate of transport related crew injury
- Use of standardized patient care handoff

colleagues[7] examined adverse events in northern Sweden. The categories of the adverse events involved transport logistics, organization, equipment/vehicle, and medical/nursing care. They were classified as a negative event, incident, risk of incident/negative event, and complaint. Given the category and classification, the risk assessment could be assigned as extreme risk, high risk, moderate risk, and low risk. The results indicated that adverse events during transport were common and often concern logistics that have little consequence. Adverse events related to medical and nursing care constituted those events of higher risk. The fundamental goal for any transport is getting the right patient with the right personnel to the right place in the right amount of time.[24] This with adequate clinical stabilization, proper and optimally functioning equipment with a safe and well maintained ambulance or aircraft for the entire transport.

SUMMARY/FUTURE OF TRANSPORT

Tremendous advances have taken place since the inception of an organized neonatal transport program in the 1940s to present day. From rudimentary incubators/isolettes to high-frequency ventilators and commercially available active cooling systems, the NICU is becoming more mobile in every sense of the word. The fundamentals of neonatal care have remained constant: temperature control, airway and respiratory management, glucose and blood pressure homeostasis, and support of the family, regardless of the technological capabilities. Highly competent and trained staff, coupled with transport-modified technology, allows for the safe and timely transport of neonates across domestic and international boundaries. A continued vigilance exists in terms of the measurement and monitoring of outcomes. Transport-based research, clinical care refinements, and ongoing robust training will only enhance the ability of the transport team in the future to continue to meet these fundamentals of care for a neonatal population at significant risk.

REFERENCES

1. Mouskou S, Troizos-Papavasileiou P, Xanthos T, et al. Neonatal transportation through the course of history. J Pediatr Neonatal Care 2015;3(1).
2. Perry S. A historical perspective on the transport of premature infants. J Obstet Gynecol Neonatal Nurs 2017;46(4):647–56.
3. Ratnavel N. Evaluating and Improving neonatal transport services. Early Hum Dev 2013;89:851–3.
4. Akula V, Gould J, Kan P, et al. Characteristics of neonatal transports in California. J Perinatol 2016;36:1122–7.
5. Campbell D, Dadiz R. Simulation in neonatal transport medicine. Semin Perinatol 2016;40:430–7.
6. Karlsen K, Trautman M, Price-Douglas W, et al. National survey of neonatal transport teams in the United States. Pediatrics 2011;128:685–91.
7. Van den Berg J, Olsson L, Svensson A, et al. Adverse events during air and ground neonatal transport: 13 years' experience from a neonatal transport team in northern Sweden. J Matern Fetal Neonatal Med 2015;28:1231–7.
8. Bastug O, Gunes T, Korkmaz L, et al. An evaluation of intrahospital transport outcomes from tertiary neonatal intensive care unit. J Matern Fetal Neonatal Med 2016;29(12):1993–8.
9. Chang A, Berry A, Jones L, et al. Specialist teams for neonatal transport to neonatal intensive care units for prevention of morbidity and mortality. Cochrane Database Syst Rev 2015;(10):CD007485.

10. Teasdale D, Hamilton C. Baby on the move: issues in neonatal transport. Paediatr Nurs 2008;20:20–5.
11. Commission on Accreditation of Medical Transport Systems (CAMTS) Available at: http://www.camts.org. Accessed December 20, 2017.
12. Commission on Accreditation of Ambulance Services Available at: www.cass.org. Accessed December 21, 2017.
13. National Alliance of Medical Transport Applications. Available at: www.naamta.com. Accessed December 23, 2017.
14. Joint Commission International. Available at: www.jointcommissioninternational.org. Accessed December 27, 2017.
15. European Aero-Medical Institute. Available at: www.eurami.org. Accessed on December 29, 2017.
16. Preventing infant death and injury during delivery. Jt Comm Perspect 2004;24(9):14–5.
17. Bruno C, Glass K. Cost-effective and low technology options for simulation and training in neonatology. Semin Perinatol 2016;40:473–9.
18. Stafford T, Hagan J, Sitler C, et al. Therapeutic hypothermia during neonatal transport: active cooling helps reach the targe. Ther Hypothermia Temp Manag 2017;7:88–94.
19. Sharakan S, Laptook AR, Ehrenkranz RA, et al. Whole body hypothermia for neonates with hypoxic ischemic encephalopathy. N Engl J Med 2005;353:1574–84.
20. Schump E, Lancaster T, Sparks D, et al. Achieving optimal therapeutic hypothermia on transport. Adv Neonatal Care 2016;16:E3–10.
21. Cotton M, Clark R. The science of neonatal high frequency ventilation. Respir Care Clin N Am 2001;7:611–31.
22. Honey G, Bleak T, Karp T, et al. Use of the Duotron transported high frequency ventilator during neonatal transport. Neonatal Netw 2007;26(3):167–74.
23. Schwartz H, Bigham M, Schoettker P, et al. Quality metrics in neonatal and pediatric critical care transport: a national Delphi project. Pediatr Crit Care Med 2015;16:711–7.
24. Schneider C, Gomez M, Lee R. Evaluation of ground ambulance, rotor wing and fixed wing aircraft services. Crit Care Clin 1992;8:533–64.

UNITED STATES POSTAL SERVICE®

Statement of Ownership, Management, and Circulation (All Periodicals Publications Except Requester Publications)

1. Publication Title	2. Publication Number	3. Filing Date
CRITICAL CARE NURSING CLINICS OF NORTH AMERICA	006 – 273	9/18/18
4. Issue Frequency	5. Number of Issues Published Annually	6. Annual Subscription Price
MAR, JUN SEP, DEC	4	$155.00

7. Complete Mailing Address of Known Office of Publication (*Not printer*) (*Street, city, county, state, and ZIP+4®*)
ELSEVIER INC.
230 Park Avenue, Suite 800
New York, NY 10169

Contact Person
STEPHEN R. BUSHING
Telephone (*Include area code*)
215-239-3688

8. Complete Mailing Address of Headquarters or General Business Office of Publisher (*Not printer*)
ELSEVIER INC.
230 Park Avenue, Suite 800
New York, NY 10169

9. Full Names and Complete Mailing Addresses of Publisher, Editor, and Managing Editor (*Do not leave blank*)

Publisher (*Name and complete mailing address*)
TAYLOR E BALL, ELSEVIER INC.
1600 JOHN F KENNEDY BLVD. SUITE 1800
PHILADELPHIA, PA 19103-2899

Editor (*Name and complete mailing address*)
KERRY HOLLAND, ELSEVIER INC.
1600 JOHN F KENNEDY BLVD. SUITE 1800
PHILADELPHIA, PA 19103-2899

Managing Editor (*Name and complete mailing address*)
PATRICK MANLEY, ELSEVIER INC.
1600 JOHN F KENNEDY BLVD. SUITE 1800
PHILADELPHIA, PA 19103-2899

10. Owner (*Do not leave blank. If the publication is owned by a corporation, give the name and address of the corporation immediately followed by the names and addresses of all stockholders owning or holding 1 percent or more of the total amount of stock. If not owned by a corporation, give the names and addresses of the individual owners. If owned by a partnership or other unincorporated firm, give its name and address as well as those of each individual owner. If the publication is published by a nonprofit organization, give its name and address.*)

Full Name	Complete Mailing Address
WHOLLY OWNED SUBSIDIARY OF REED/ELSEVIER, US HOLDINGS	1600 JOHN F KENNEDY BLVD. SUITE 1800 PHILADELPHIA, PA 19103-2899

11. Known Bondholders, Mortgagees, and Other Security Holders Owning or Holding 1 Percent or More of Total Amount of Bonds, Mortgages, or Other Securities. If none, check box → ☐ None

Full Name	Complete Mailing Address
N/A	

12. Tax Status (*For completion by nonprofit organizations authorized to mail at nonprofit rates*) (*Check one*)
The purpose, function, and nonprofit status of this organization and the exempt status for federal income tax purposes:
☒ Has Not Changed During Preceding 12 Months
☐ Has Changed During Preceding 12 Months (*Publisher must submit explanation of change with this statement*)

PS Form **3526**, July 2014 *[Page 1 of 4 (see instructions page 4)]* PSN: 7530-01-000-9931 **PRIVACY NOTICE:** See our privacy policy on *www.usps.com.*

13. Publication Title		14. Issue Date for Circulation Data Below	
CRITICAL CARE NURSING CLINICS OF NORTH AMERICA		JUNE 2018	
15. Extent and Nature of Circulation		**Average No. Copies Each Issue During Preceding 12 Months**	**No. Copies of Single Issue Published Nearest to Filing Date**
a. Total Number of Copies (*Net press run*)		167	214
b. Paid Circulation (*By Mail and Outside the Mail*)	(1) Mailed Outside-County Paid Subscriptions Stated on PS Form 3541 (*Include paid distribution above nominal rate, advertiser's proof copies, and exchange copies*)	84	96
	(2) Mailed In-County Paid Subscriptions Stated on PS Form 3541 (*Include paid distribution above nominal rate, advertiser's proof copies, and exchange copies*)	0	0
	(3) Paid Distribution Outside the Mails Including Sales Through Dealers and Carriers, Street Vendors, Counter Sales, and Other Paid Distribution Outside USPS®	28	37
	(4) Paid Distribution by Other Classes of Mail Through the USPS (e.g., First-Class Mail®)	0	0
c. Total Paid Distribution (*Sum of 15b (1), (2), (3), and (4)*) ▶		112	133
d. Free or Nominal Rate Distribution (*By Mail and Outside the Mail*)	(1) Free or Nominal Rate Outside-County Copies included on PS Form 3541	46	65
	(2) Free or Nominal Rate In-County Copies Included on PS Form 3541	0	0
	(3) Free or Nominal Rate Copies Mailed at Other Classes Through the USPS (e.g., First-Class Mail)	0	0
	(4) Free or Nominal Rate Distribution Outside the Mail (*Carriers or other means*)	0	0
e. Total Free or Nominal Rate Distribution (*Sum of 15d (1), (2), (3) and (4)*)		46	65
f. Total Distribution (*Sum of 15c and 15e*) ▶		158	198
g. Copies not Distributed (*See Instructions to Publishers #4 (page #3)*) ▶		9	16
h. Total (*Sum of 15f and g*)		167	214
i. Percent Paid (*15c divided by 15f times 100*) ▶		70.89%	67.17%

* If you are claiming electronic copies, go to line 16 on page 3. If you are not claiming electronic copies, skip to line 17 on page 3.

16. Electronic Copy Circulation	**Average No. Copies Each Issue During Preceding 12 Months**	**No. Copies of Single Issue Published Nearest to Filing Date**
a. Paid Electronic Copies ▶	0	0
b. Total Paid Print Copies (Line 15c) + Paid Electronic Copies (Line 16a) ▶	112	133
c. Total Print Distribution (Line 15f) + Paid Electronic Copies (Line 16a) ▶	158	198
d. Percent Paid (Both Print & Electronic Copies) (16b divided by 16c × 100) ▶	70.89%	67.17%

☒ **I certify that 50% of all my distributed copies (electronic and print) are paid above a nominal price.**

17. Publication of Statement of Ownership

☒ If the publication is a general publication, publication of this statement is required. Will be printed in the DECEMBER 2018 issue of this publication. ☐ Publication not required.

18. Signature and Title of Editor, Publisher, Business Manager, or Owner
STEPHEN R. BUSHING - INVENTORY DISTRIBUTION CONTROL MANAGER
Date: 9/18/18

I certify that all information furnished on this form is true and complete. I understand that anyone who furnishes false or misleading information on this form or who omits material or information requested on the form may be subject to criminal sanctions (including fines and imprisonment) and/or civil sanctions (including civil penalties).

PS Form **3526**, July 2014 (*Page 3 of 4*) **PRIVACY NOTICE:** See our privacy policy on *www.usps.com.*

Printed and bound by CPI Group (UK) Ltd, Croydon, CR0 4YY
07/10/2024
01040506-0014